COACH YOURSELF
TO HEALTH
AND HAPPINESS

The

POCKET
LIFE
COACH

Pete Chapman

Crown House Publishing Limited

D0277866

First published by

Crown House Publishing Ltd
Crown Buildings, Bancyfelin, Carmarthen, Wales, SA33 5ND, UK
www.crownhouse.co.uk

and

Crown House Publishing Company LLC
6 Trowbridge Drive, Suite 5, Bethel, CT 06801, USA
www.chpus.com

British Library of Cataloguing-in-Publication Data
A catalogue entry for this book is available
from the British Library.

13-digit ISBN 978-184590071-7

LCCN 2007928041

Edited by Fiona Spencer Thomas
Printed and bound in the UK by
The Cromwell Press, Trowbridge, Wiltshire

CONTENTS

INTRODUCTION

Have you ever had a dream hangover? "What's one of those?" I sense you ask? Well, it's that sinking feeling you get when you wake up from a really nice dream, where life is so much more satisfying, free and easy, and you have seemingly unlimited powers of skill and confidence. This contrasts starkly with the cold light and reality of the dawn of another day in your real life. Damn those sweet dreams, we enjoy them at the time, but they don't half match up poorly with reality sometimes. It often happens the other way around of course, when you have a nightmare and it's such a relief to wake up and find out you are not chained to a desk in a burning office building or sentenced by a judge, who looks remarkably like your mother-in-law, to a lifetime of watching paint dry on the walls of a beautiful city that you have been banished from for ever.

Dreams are powerful things. They are part of our everyday experience. We are glad when the bad ones don't come true and we are sad when, each day we awake to find that we seem to be getting no closer to making the good ones a reality. Sometimes dreams do come true, small ones and big ones, good ones and not so good ones. We do seem to have the capacity to turn imagination and fantasy into our reality. These dreams are slightly different, I know, as they are deep desires and hopes from the heart, but I'm sure you get the message. Deep in our psyches we have many hopes and fears, and these often show themselves in strange dramas that play out while we are sleeping, coming to life, as it were. Sometimes though, they can jump out of our dreams and into our daily life too.

We seem to have the capacity to bring our imagination to life. Many people do this in a negative way without knowing how or why we do so, but we often end up feeling unlucky or blighted in life. We soon start to expect the worst. Some people, on the other hand, just seem to be blessed with the Midas Touch. One day they get an idea, a flash of inspiration, and soon there is a successful new business venture under way, or they seem to be able to find new ways to improve their relationships, bodies or lifestyle when they need to.

Other people seem to be able to just conjure up whatever they want and 'poof', as if by magic, it goes from fantasy to a new reality. The question is, Can anyone do it? The message of this book is, yes, absolutely we can. Routinely we all manifest our dreams and hopes as well as, unfortunately, our fears. Most of us don't know just how we do it. We are truly creative machines, we just have to learn how to create a life more akin to our aspirations. It is definitely easy to create, we do it every day with our choices and will, but it is not always so easy to change the way we create.

This book is about how to bring your true desires, talents, powers and purpose out of your head and into your life and stop the cycle of creating problems, drama, difficulty and illness. It is about understanding what potential you have and how to develop it, recognising and overcoming limitations, fears and recurring obstacles; freeing yourself up to be the best you can. We all have a better self inside. We all have a better life to live, and we all have this potential waiting to be unveiled.

Life can often seem like a scene from a western where the hero is dragged along behind the wild horse through mud and cacti, winding up battered and bruised in a strange place surrounded by a hostile crowd. Other times it feels like smooth sailing, sunny and calm, where the slightest whim is granted and the smell of roses is the order of the day. The skill is in turning low and negative expectations into high and positive ones, problems into solutions, illness into vitality and tragic drama into romantic comedy. The objective of this book is to create a map of all the known lands in the world of human potential and to illuminate a secure path through the minefield of life's imposed and self-imposed obstacles. It is a path only you can tread but one that you can get help to locate and navigate. There is such a thing as potential, a best possible scenario, and we all have the ability to make the best of what we have been given. Dreams can become reality and we all have the ability to manifest our hearts' desires. Ordinary people just like you and I do extraordinary things every day, things that they only initially 'dreamed of', but eventually lived out.

However possible our goals and dreams and desired changes may be, it doesn't necessarily mean they appear in front of you immediately with the wave of your magic wand. There are a lot of pieces to this puzzle. Change requires strength. Yes, we need instruction and method but we get nowhere without passion, drive, courage and perseverance. The kind of creativity and change we are talking about, the power to transform a life, a body, an attitude, a future, requires the kind of strength, imagination and application that you may have thought only other people had, but not you. So many of us give up on our goals and dreams and sometimes even the merest hope of positive change because we cannot sustain the focus and confidence we need to make it all happen. It is certainly not the norm to act and think this way but it is becoming more widespread, as people everywhere and from every walk of life are demanding health, happiness, independence and freedom for themselves and their families.

We all have the potential to live healthy and consistently joyous lives. All the resources are there. The only thing stopping us is ourselves; a part conditioned, part self-created programming that determines how we think, what we believe to be true about ourselves and our world, and what to expect from our future. For many of us at the moment, that programming is negative and limiting, but it certainly doesn't have to be. We think we don't have the strength but we do. We may not always have had the know-how but, if the desire and the will are there, the way is surely not far behind. For many of us, our story, the one we star in every day, may need a rewrite. Maybe it won't be a drastic one but, all the same, it begins with an appreciation that we ourselves are the playwrights and that we do indeed have the power, however hidden it might be, to get the job done. But what is that job? What are the changes that need to be made? What are the talents waiting to spring forth? This is all up to you to decide, of course, but this book aims to give you the insight and the strength to make the necessary changes, whatever they may be. You are the one steering the ship, as it were. You have to decide on the direction. Who are you really? What is the best version of you and what are you supposed to be doing with the gifts of body, mind and life that you have been given? For these are gifts, and quite a responsibility.

Each of our lives affects many others around us. When setting the course and as we search our hearts for exactly what is desired, we need to remember what is important. Is the new convertible more important than a healthy body? Is a new career more important than a happy family? Which comes first, love or money? Can we have both? Can we have it all? As the voiceover guy says: "These questions and more will be answered shortly." But for now, yes, I believe we can have it all. We just need to know how to develop our strengths and powers and then how to create our reality. If we are fit, flexible, focused, free, fun-loving and prepared to take a risk, we will no doubt find what it is that we are looking for.

When do we know that we have it? Ah, that is the real question. Wellbeing, creativity and happiness can be taught but only the owner of the body, mind and life can appreciate and accept it. Only we can know when we are full when that time comes. Begin with an attitude of humility, appreciation, open-mindedness and courage and you are well on your way. This book is just a prop on the stage of this act of your life. It is up to you how the play continues from this moment on. Break a leg!

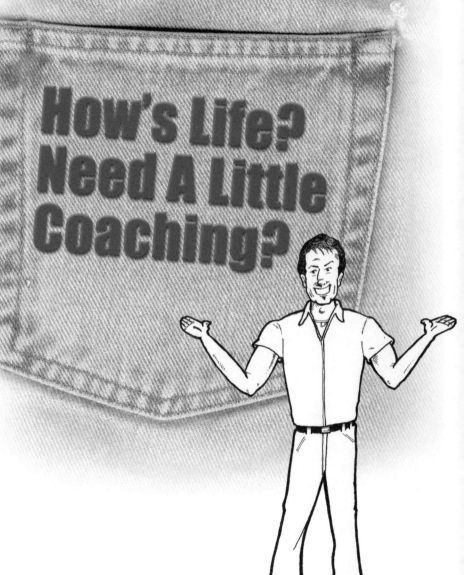

CHAPTER ONE

How's Life? Need A Little Coaching?

LIFE COACH YOURSELF TO HEALTH AND HAPPINESS

None of us has all the answers all of the time, especially when it comes to our own life. We all need a little objective guidance from time to time when we want to improve or change something about ourselves and our lives. It is not always so easy to find someone who has the ability to help us change for the better. Sometimes it's a money issue and sometimes it's a privacy issue or possibly a lack of motivation. Sometimes we give up trying to make things better and allow our dreams gradually to fade away while we make do with an inferior quality of health and lifestyle. One thing is for sure though, no one is going to do it for us; we have to find the will as well as the way to get ourselves there.

Not everyone would automatically think of a life coach as an option or resource to help one overcome limitations and sticking points and provide the inspiration and guidance that we are talking about. Many people are not fully aware of what life coaching even is or what a life coach can do for them. Granted, each life coach has their own style but generally it is a very modern concept and job description that incorporates many existing and traditional sources of help such as psychology, spiritual guidance, careers counselling, personal training, time management and mentoring. The aim of this particular book is to help you, the reader realise your potential, physically and mentally, and find the greatest success possible, whatever that might be. The idea here, is that when we are organised and focused, free from negativity and hang-ups and living a balanced and healthy life, then we are so much more productive, relaxed, creative and purposeful. So, simply put, life coaching is about empowering people. If your goal is to improve your health, your prospects, your relationships, your image and your life experience, then you have found what you are looking for.

This workbook is your tool, your personal life coach as it were, to help you rediscover the healthiest, most productive, positive and creative you. It is up to you to use it well. Have a look again at the Contents page. It lists the main areas that you will be addressing as you work on improving yourself holistically (in all the ways you need to). This is your guide but you can do it all yourself. It is easier than you think to achieve these things and get closer than you ever thought possible to your true potential. All you need is a map, a tool and some energy. Each person reading this has their own goals in mind and their own problems to overcome. You may be in need of a complete reinvention. You may be trying to get over a major trauma or loss and trying to build up your life again. You may have a chronic health condition that you haven't been able to overcome. You might just feel as though you are in a rut and that it is time for a shake-up, a change, a lifestyle make-over perhaps. Either way this is a great opportunity to do a little soul searching, get to know yourself better, remind yourself what you are capable of and work on yourself to be the best you can. We all need to do this at times so that we don't lose track of our goals and dreams and the things that are most important to us.

It is completely natural to want to be better and improve. It is completely natural to strive to progress, improve and adapt. This is how evolution works. We are no different from other creatures in that we must evolve and improve regularly if we are to survive and prosper in an ever-changing world. As nature strives to find the best way so must we. Our best is wrapped up in our potential waiting to be unfurled and expressed but so often our lifestyles become our masters rather than the other way around. It is time to take charge of our lives again. All achievement and potential happiness starts with us; with a desire and a decision. Do you want the best for yourself and those around you or is mere existence and a so-so life good enough for you? This is YOUR LIFE, live it the best way you can.

USING YOUR POCKET LIFE COACH

This book covers a lot of topics so don't rush through it, take your time. Read a section, think about it and come back to it later. It will sink in better that way. There are sections for guidance and instruction and some that are just intended to inspire you and provoke reflection. Work through the book steadily and fill in the sections that require you to. You will become more aware than ever of your true current situation, how you spend your time, how you think, your beliefs about yourself and the world around you, what you eat, what activities you participate in, generally how you live this life at the moment. All of this determines who you are today and what your quality of life is going to be tomorrow.

Once you have a clear picture of what is really going on now in your body, mind and your life, then you are in a position to make lasting changes. The workbook-like nature of this programme is just how it would be if you had a real life coach working with you. You would be asked to evaluate just how you live your life currently and then you would be given options to improve all important aspects and then methods to apply these changes to your current schedule and routine. So if you want the best results, use this book to its fullest extent. Remember Rome wasn't built in a day so be patient yet determined. Once you have read and completed all the sections, then it is just a matter of living your life with a little more balance and consideration of what is healthy and good for you.

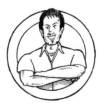

I am your Pocket Life Coach, your partner to help you use the tools in this book. Remember you are the driving force and it is up to you, as always, to learn what you can and make the necessary changes as best you can. Take it one day and one aspect of your life at a time. Good luck.

LET'S BE HONEST NOW, SHALL WE?

Before you can change anything you must be able to understand where you are at the moment. When you overhaul your financial plan you look at exactly what you spend and what you earn. Then you make decisions based on your actual situation compared to your ideal situation. For the best results in any endeavour we always have to find our starting point, our actual position now so that we can plan ahead with confidence. Many problems in life are caused by our reluctance to be realistic and honest with ourselves and to face up to our situations realistically instead of viewing our world in a way that makes us feel better temporarily. This view is often unrealistic and it boils down to a lack of honesty on our part. The famous movie line "You can't handle the truth," underlines the fear many of us have about looking closely at what is actually going on. You see we have each developed standards relative to what we believe to be good, fair and correct. When we really start to be honest with ourselves and look at the way we really live and think, so many of the causes of our pain and disappointment show themselves. We spend far too much time papering over the cracks of our reality with what amounts to storytelling and self-delusion. Likewise, sometimes we are over critical of ourselves when, in fact, that is not a fair and true evaluation either. If you are serious about changing your current situation you have to find out what the reality of it is. This true picture may take a while to put together but again, with practice it is something that you can accomplish and with this powerful knowledge you can move forward from a stable starting point.

Once you have established a clear view of your world, you are in a much more powerful position to effect change and recognise problem conditions that may need to be altered. You will also be able to identify those things that you previously thought needed changing which are in fact, perfectly acceptable. It is all about saving you time and energy, being more efficient by making your starting point your ultimate source of power. It is the place to strike from and retreat safely back to, and it is so important to identify it before you make any move to better yourself. There is no point in working towards an ideal situation until you are aware of your current and actual position. Bite the bullet and face facts while being kind to yourself along the way. You will be glad you did.

WHAT IS YOUR BEST? DEFINING YOUR POTENTIAL

This is the dictionary definition of the word potential: capable of being but not yet in existence; latent; having possibility, capability or power. Everything created has its own potential, an ideal, a best case scenario, as it were. This book attempts to define what this word means when associated with us, yes, even you. The reason we need this is that, once a definition has been established, then it is just a matter of the application process. Easy right?

We would all love to realise our true potential, get our bodies into the best condition possible, to train and develop our minds into a powerful thinking, problem solving and creative force. We all want to be as happy, fulfilled and free as possible. Yet if it were that easy, then we would all have it wouldn't we? We know it isn't easy to achieve our best and this may be due largely to the fact that very few of us know what is our best potential state or what is required to achieve it.

To begin the definition process for human potential, it may be easier to learn from those who have mastered it. Legend tells of a few who have personified perfection and completion in every way. We are inspired by these 'super humans' but we don't always feel as though we have the same capabilities or potential that they had. We need more relevant and up-to-date advice on how to make changes and improvements while we live this hectic life of ours. Although legendary characters inspire, we still have to apply their ideals to today's lifestyles. Our potential hasn't actually changed but our culture and lifestyle has, and methods and techniques must keep up. It seems a good time to redefine potential and remind ourselves what we are capable of in a world with so much ill health, antisocial behaviour, fear and uncertainty. Time for a new approach perhaps?

We all have amazing potential, but generally we operate at far less than our capabilities. We have an abundance of powers and skills, some known and previously acquired and now lost, some known but never developed, others unknown and lying latent, waiting to be ignited, animated and expressed. Each moment of each day we operate on a particular level somewhere below our capabilities. In general our health and vitality is not what it could be. Our bodies are more tired and polluted than ever, our minds more narrow, scattered and prone to negativity and our spirits yearn for beauty, purpose, passion and freedom. We have lost touch with our more powerful, loving and authentic selves.

Long ago we were much more aware of our powers because we lived closer to nature and knew what was required to stay fit and strong. Our survival and our ability to produce strong and healthy offspring were paramount. Now life is relatively safe and most of our demanding and dangerous tasks are performed by machines. Because of this we seem to have lost some of our natural strengths, skills and instincts. We have largely forgotten what we really need and what we are here for so we have become detached from an understanding of our own potential. It is time to realise, once again, what we are truly capable of being. This book will attempt to remind you of these things and help you to apply them to your daily life.

Our potential is laid out in our DNA programming and it dictates what we need to function properly. With an animal-like knowing our instincts used to tell us what to do, what was good or bad for us. Now we have to relearn how to sharpen them and reconnect with our inner voice of wisdom. We know, deep within us how to be our best. We just need a little reminding and to be provided with a few methods so that we can apply this wisdom to our daily lives. It won't take long, let's start now.

CHAPTER TWO

Making the Best Of It. A Better Life

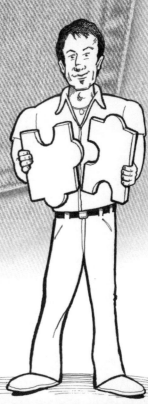

THE PUZZLE OF LIFE

We all have the potential to have a great life but it is up to us to make it happen. Life is like a picture made up of pieces just like a jigsaw puzzle. When we get all the pieces and put them together in their right places we see and appreciate the complete picture. The way we live our lives and the choices we make determine what kind of picture we create and it depends on the pieces we put into it. To be prepared for life we must know what is good for us (the pieces) and how to organise our time so that we can put in the pieces in the right way. This way we ensure that we get the most out it because we have put into it the best that we can. It's simple. The more of our needs we have met in our life (pieces of the puzzle), the happier, healthier and more successful we are. These are the more important pieces of the puzzle.

Your mind needs:

1. Progress – We don't need perfection just progress. Try to see some progress and achievement (however small) each week.

2. Goals – Set realistic ones, keep them up-to-date, and review them regularly.

3. Organisation – Plan the next day the evening before.

4. Problems/Challenge – This is how you grow and learn.

5. Achievement – We all need to feel useful and productive.

6. Reading and Learning – Expand your mind like a muscle. Read regularly. Learn a new skill.

7. Rules and Boundaries – Sometimes we need to be disciplined in our lives so that we can contain and focus our energies and perform at our best.

8. Relaxation – As much as the mind needs to be worked, it also needs to relax and stop thinking. Learn to be passive sometimes and take time out regularly.

(see the Healthy Mind section on pages 90–93 for full list)

Your body needs:

1. **Oxygen** – Oxygen heals and revitalises the body and mind. Exercise and breathing exercises are required regularly.

2. **Water** – You need a minimum of eight glasses per day.

3. **Nutrition** – Three nutritious meals and a snack per day.

4. **Sleep** – Seven to nine hours depending on your body. Relaxation and stretching before bed helps restful sleep.

5. **Exercise** – More than necessary for the maintenance of physical abilities and energy flow, a celebration of being fit and alive!

6. **Stretching** – Good health depends on good posture and being free of muscular tension.

7. **Hygiene** – Keep yourself and your environment clean for good health.

8. **Touch/Hugs/Massage** – It's all good. Make it loving and fun!

    (see body section on pages 50–51 for rest of list)

Your inner self needs:

1. **Inspiration** – Seek out regular inspiration, books, music, church, friends and mentors. We all need a boost.

2   **Appreciation** – Appreciate what you have, everything is a gift.

3. **Truth** – Be honest with yourself and others – you will be rewarded. Stand in your own truth and you will be empowered.

4. **Freedom** – Don't get tied down too much. Along with your health, your freedom of choice is your greatest asset.

5. **Laughter/Fun** – Be light and don't take life too seriously. Try to laugh and have fun every day.

6. **Friends/Family/Love** – We all need love and support. The more you love yourself, the more love you will receive.

7. **Forgiveness** – Release your negative pain by forgiving yourself and others for their mistakes. Your health suffers greatly from carrying this burden around.

8. **Nature/Beauty** – Food for the soul. All of Creation is beautiful and we are all connected.

9. **Hope** – When all hope is lost, so are we.

   (see spirituality section on pages 127–129 for full list)

Missing Pieces

Our problems begin when we live out of balance, make poor choices and manage our time badly so that some of the pieces of that puzzle are missing. Some are felt more than others such as the basics like good nutrition, water and sleep. We can get away with missing pieces some of the time, but if we want to be really happy and healthy and realise our potential, we must try to complete the picture. Our missing needs create a kind of void which, because we live twenty-four hours a day, will be filled by something. That something is usually an excess of some kind like too much work, food, TV, computers or booze or other things. So it is not necessarily what we do that harms us, it is what we don't do that creates the space for excess, obsession and addiction. So the message here is this; Do something new, needed and positive instead of too much of the same old thing! The more needs we miss regularly, the less balanced, healthy, productive, patient and loving we are. We also become more susceptible to stress, negative thinking and illness and this, in turn, leads to more unhelpful choices. This is how we 'create' our own difficulties and problems much of the time.

WELLBEING, IMMUNITY AND LONGEVITY

Along with an outline of our potential, this book attempts to define a general recipe for optimum wellbeing that fits us all. We are all human beings and, as such, we have our requirements to function at our best just like all living things. And not just living things. It is the same way even with machines. If you don't maintain a mechanical object, it too will perform poorly and is liable to break down prematurely. We too need to be maintained but we need more than that. We need to grow, become fitter and more dynamic so that we can take on all that life has to offer. The closer we get to achieving this state of balance and strength, the more resilient our immune systems become and the more smoothly our bodies perform. This not only translates into a better quality of life, but a longer and happier life.

This sounds simple, and it is, but we make life difficult for ourselves because of our choices. We often get distracted from what we know is good for us and forget the things we need to do to get our health and vitality back up again. So, in addition to this book being a guide to your wellbeing and personal potential it is also a roadmap to guide you back to health if you have mislaid it somewhere along life's rocky highway. It can serve as a self-healing system, if you like. Whatever your shortcoming or problem, you must believe that your natural and true state of wellbeing and vitality is waiting to be rediscovered. It is just a matter of returning to the balance you need and getting your crucial requirements met. Only you can really heal yourself because, ultimately, it is down to you and your choices. You are mainly responsible for your health as well as your longevity. The choices you make, the way you spend your time, directly affect the state of your relative health and happiness.

We all have to find our own way towards wellness and fulfillment. Some of us just need a little more guidance than others. You may just have a key to a better future now. So what is it going to be? Are you going to accept it, use it and live it? Or are you going to let another opportunity for growth and genuine progress slip by? The choice is yours, as always.

BALANCED LIVING

Balance is strength, a sure footing for success. A healthy life is a balanced life. Balance in the context of health means living your life in a way that meets your needs holistically, i.e. mentally, physically and emotionally; creating an environment for optimum wellbeing, vitality and fulfillment. How we spend our time and our general attitude to life, determines our state of balance and wellbeing. Unfortunately, we often live life out of balance. With a lack of basic knowledge, busy schedules, pressures and distractions we miss out on doing some of the things which are vital for maintaining our wellbeing. We need to get back to living in balance to make sure that our life is not only healthy and sustainable but also fulfilling. The simple way to check is to look at the list of needs and see how many you are missing out on regularly. Some will be more important than others such as drinking enough water, eating good food or getting sufficient exercise or relaxation. You may be spending too much time on some things like TV or boozing in the pub instead of reading or outdoor pursuits. There is a time for everything. It is just a matter of knowing what things need to be accounted for in your schedule and then planning accordingly. The message here is; Get what you need, find your natural balance and return to your better self. You will find life easier and more fun!

Work/Life Balance

It is not always easy in a busy life full of demands on our time and resources to know the best way to divide and manage our time. The upcoming section on time management should help you begin the process of organising your time as best as you can. Let's start with a few basic ideas. We know we need to sleep for eight hours a night or a third of our lives. Sleep is one of our most important needs. This leaves two thirds or sixteen hours a day to do with what we wish, or think we should do, or have to do. It is impossible to satisfy all our needs by working all the time and equally impossible to do the same if you are playing and relaxing. So we do have to figure out some way to balance all this up. We struggle to make sense of life today because we can't find the balance between these three major elements of our lives and continue to spend excessive time on what we think we should be doing, and not what we 'need' to be doing for our wellbeing.

We all need to work and feel accomplished and worthy. Just ask lottery winners if they are really any happier for retiring too early. Without working and making an effort, we don't enjoy our free time and leisure as much. We can't have one without the other because they both provide us with our needs. What we have to do is create a schedule where we get all our obligations and work done as well as have adequate time to get the rest of our needs met. Again, balance and sensible time management is required. Basically wellbeing and genuine life fulfillment is dependent on how you spend your time and the choices you make.

If we look at life as a balance of working or effort, playing or leisure time and resting or sleeping, we should be spending an equal amount of time on each of these aspects. Together, they provide all the different pieces of the jigsaw for a healthy, happy and fulfilling life. When we do too much of one thing, something else suffers. Some days we spend more time working and some days we miss sleep but if we aim to make up the time by the end of each week, then our health and general wellbeing will be so much better. Just take a few moments now to evaluate whether your current lifestyle satisfies your needs or not. Once you have identified the elements that are missing

Most Absent Needs	Others to Watch

regularly, you can begin the process of organising your time so that they can be brought back in and the balance restored.

STRESS MANAGEMENT

God promises a safe landing but not a calm passage

Bulgarian Proverb

As we learn to make changes and put together a new, healthier and fulfilling lifestyle, we have to learn to deal with stress better. Stress is the wear and tear our bodies experience as we adjust to our continually changing environment. Stress affects us physically and mentally as well as emotionally. It can create positive as well as negative feelings and reactions. As a positive influence, stress can help compel us to action, resulting in new accomplishments, needed change and an exciting new perspective. As a negative influence, it can result in feelings of distrust, rejection, anger and depression, which in turn can lead to health problems such as headaches, upset stomach, rashes, insomnia, ulcers, high blood pressure and more. With the birth of a baby, moving house, a job promotion, a new relationship or the death of a loved one, for example, we experience stress as we readjust our lives. In so adjusting to different circumstances, stress will help or hinder us depending on how we react to it. The proverb 'Pray not for a lighter load, but for stronger shoulders' best describes the attitude we need to have in order to maintain our strength and cope with our challenges. When we are organised, fit and healthy, focused and relaxed, we are in the best position to manage stressful situations. In this balanced and content state we generally create fewer problems for ourselves and deal better with those that inevitably arise from a life full of challenge and change.

 To help you manage your stress better, here are a few tips to ease the pressure:

- Don't take everything too seriously all the time

- Don't make promises you cannot keep

- Don't always take things so personally

- Take a few deep breaths and extra time before making a decision in a stressful situation

- Get enough sleep. It's hard to think straight when you're tired

- Make sure you have enough energy to cope, eat a good meal and get some rest and then act

- Look at your diet. Try to cut down on the meats and processed foods, caffeine, alcohol and other stimulants. Eat as clean, healthy and fresh as you can

- Ask for help a little more

- Don't rely so much on others when you can do things yourself

- Compartmentalise work and private time

- Use your sense of humour. Laugh at yourself a little more

- Remember, your problem isn't the only one in the world

- Try not to judge others until you have all the facts

- Face up to the decisions you have to make

- Try to view things with compassionate eyes and an open heart and mind

- Believe in your strength and ability to cope

- Stay in your truth, trust yourself

- Are you putting too much pressure on yourself?

- Try to remain in the present more and think of what can be done now instead of worrying about what might happen in the future

- You are NOT your problems. Learn to detach from them once you have done your best to make things better

- Have you created the problem yourself? Can you 'un-create' it? Try to make life a little easier on yourself and the people around you by creating less drama

- Learn more about the subject that is giving you problems

- Try to see the subject from ALL sides

- Sleep on your decisions when you can and give the problem to a higher power while you sleep

- Stretch and relax each evening. De-stress with exercise. Take a nice walk in nature regularly

- Do you laugh enough? Put on your favourite funny movie or spend some time with a friend who makes you giggle. Laughing is the best kind of stress relief

- Try a natural herbal stress reliever like St John's Wort, Kava or Valerian root if taking herbs is OK with you

- Take a dance or yoga class or try a new hobby

After a Hard Day

You will help yourself so much if you can get into the habit of taking a small amount of time at the end of your working day to exercise, stretch out or meditate away your tensions. Just 10–15 minutes is enough to act as an effective and necessary buffer between your world of obligations and your free, leisure time. If you don't shake off the tension then it will follow you into the evening and even on to the next day. This way it accumulates and it is only a matter of time until you have stress related disorders and problems. Take time to let go and refresh yourself. Maybe, once you have de-stressed, the perfect thing you need is a good old hobby to look forward to, probably not on-line gambling but something a little healthier maybe! As always, it's up to you.

Money and Stress

If you haven't got money, be nice

Danish Proverb

Money can be a wonderful source of freedom and creativity but it can also be a tremendous stress. Remember that money is a tool and although we need it, we don't need as many things as we think we do. When you start making the distinctions between wants and genuine needs you will save yourself a lot of unnecessary expense and unwanted stress. Be on top of your money not underneath it. Keep track of all your expenses whether they are made in cash or credit, debit or cheques. This will ensure you not only don't overspend but also show you exactly what your spending habits are (just like a diet journal tells you exactly what you are putting into your mouth) so that you can make adjustments in the future. This will help you to come to terms with the reality of your relationship with money.

 Are You Spending Money You Don't Have?

Money and Happiness

Every day in life you are tested. You know the phrase 'what goes around, comes around'? This is your karma. 'As ye sow so shall ye reap' is another of those old phrases giving us the lesson that we must tread lightly and be considerate as we go about our daily lives. If we want to be peaceful and fortunate, we must be prepared to be honest, not greedy, and be more kind, generous and considerate of others. Whenever we go against this and act for purely selfish reasons, then we cause ourselves problems by creating bad energy or negative karma around us. Money is always a good test for our karma. There are so many opportunities for us to 'smash and grab' without considering the consequences but this way of living is very short sighted. We never get away with wrongdoing, even when we think we have. Nature and life in general has a way of finding balance and justice and we cannot escape these rules as much as we think we can. When we get greedy we lose out in the end. When we are selfish we only shoot ourselves in the foot because we are attracting more bad energy as a reflection of what we are 'sowing'. When we consider the impact of our actions, we keep a 'clean slate' with our karma and have faith that our hard work will be rewarded and we will have all the abundance we need. Remember, wealth is a state of mind. Be happy with what you have while you work in balance to give yourself more freedom by using the tool called money for the benefit of yourself and others. Take a little time to write out a budget for yourself. You will see what money you are really making and spending and then you can decide if you need to make any changes in this department. As always with evaluation, be realistic and consider what is really good for you.

PET PROJECTS

Not all of us have the perfect job where we are able to express our range of skills, talents and passions. This is why we need 'pet projects' or hobbies and purposeful pastimes to feel happy and fulfilled. We all have a creative side or a desire to express something and develop ourselves further but it is not always easy to find the time or energy for these things that so enrich our lives. However, with good organisation and time management, most of us can and should fit a favourite project into our schedules. Here are some examples that are good for expanding your mind and horizons:

1. Volunteer Work

2. Playing a Musical Instrument

3. Arts and Crafts

4. Side Business

5. Mentor Programme

6. Community Involvement

7. Home Improvement

8. Learning a New Language

9. Self Help Reading

If you have a really busy schedule, children or other commitments, maybe your favourite project is to just take some quiet time to read, go for a walk or just have some peace and quiet. Remember it is important to try actively to be fulfilled but sometimes it is right to just do nothing and be passive. Organise your time and resources and maybe you can find space in your life for an interesting hobby as well as that quiet time. The idea is to do something you like, do it as well as you can and enjoy the accomplishment as well as the added social involvement with other like-minded people.

THE POWER OF WORK

Simply put; we are what we do and what we think. To find out who we are, people ask us what we do. We reply by telling them what we do to earn a living but this is a limited definition. We define ourselves by our work even though we spend roughly only a third of our lives doing it. But to be happy and fulfilled, it is vitally important that we find satisfaction in our working lives so that, whatever it is we do for a living, we find as much satisfaction and reward as possible from this time. I believe we can only do this by adopting a positive attitude to work as well as ensuring that we are as organised, prepared, fit and as healthy as possible. This is why this programme puts so much emphasis on setting up effective time management, goal setting and positive thinking strategies.

Briefly here I want to make a quick statement about our working practices and attitude. There is no doubt that, in reality, we can get as much pleasure and satisfaction from our work time as we do from our play time. All you have to do is look at your needs and see how stimulating and fulfilling work and the accomplishments derived from it can bring. When it comes to realising our true potential, or realising any goal for that matter, we all know that we have to work for it. Life is a never ending process of problem solving, goal setting, effort, challenge and achievement. It is only after we have put out that we can expect to get back, so the way we view our work and the way we do our work is key to our overall wellbeing. We can never be truly fulfilled while we hate or resent our work. We have to develop a joy and appreciation of work if we are fully to appreciate everything that it has to offer us. Some of the benefits are more subtle than the obvious ones of monetary reward and status. There are so many hidden benefits to spending our work time well that can never be underestimated. Our natural lazy tendencies encourage us to take short cuts and yearn for retirement but if we keep a good work/life balance, find satisfaction in our job and the other areas of our lives, we should reap the benefits of our accomplishments till our dying days. Having said all that, we can never forget that balance must never be forsaken as we manage our time and lives. While we must try to give our all while we are at work, we have to ensure that we train ourselves mentally and physically to be strong and focused as well as relaxed and dynamic. We must also be careful not to overwork and cut too heavily into our rest and leisure time. The messages here are clear; Work to live, do not live to work; Work smart as well as hard; Be organised and prepared; Enjoy your accomplishments and appreciate your past achievements. Our work should not define us completely but it should give us the resources, skills and confidence to realise our potential and be the happiest we can be.

ACTIVE AND PASSIVE LIVING

You have already read about our need to be balanced and this concept emerges yet again. Indeed, much of this book is about the active things you can do to realise your potential, after all, this is an instructional tool first and foremost. In any working system, and our bodies and minds are no different, one must include down time; rest, peace, calm and passivity. Today so much is made of what we should be doing to live a good life, but sometimes we just need to do nothing, be still, breathe; just be. It is fairly difficult, to say the least, for some of us to be inactive. It is considered by many to be dead time instead of down time. This couldn't be more wrong.

If the opposite of active is passive, then we should spend equal time on activity as we do being passive. This doesn't mean lying around comatose during the day; it means taking the time to be quiet if you can, maybe after a meal or for a few minutes in the morning before the mayhem of the day begins. It means letting things happen and come to you instead of pushing all the time. Any good salesman will tell you that sometimes you just have to wait and let the results of your efforts come back to you. Sometimes less really is more. Life is not a race, it is a voyage and you need to take frequent stops along the way if you are to realise your ultimate destination. Good, restful sleep, quiet meditation, reading, music, nature, even a little well chosen TV is good sometimes, all this is needed to balance out the obligations and pressures of modern living. Don't feel guilty about allowing yourself this time. It is necessary for you to be at your best, smiling, enthusiastic and patient. Don't short change yourself with your passive time. This may not seem too realistic for some of you who seem to have no time to spare at all. The Time Management section will give you a few tips on how to create and maximise your time. With a little planning and setting a few boundaries, efficient working practices and good physical energy levels, you can definitely reap the huge benefits of more passive and quiet time.

CHAPTER THREE

Beginning the Changes. Some Useful Tools

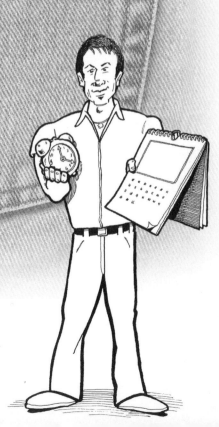

MOTIVATION

Whether you think you can or think you can't, you're right

Henry Ford

Motivation really boils down to how much we are prepared to put into something, how much we want it. To achieve our goals and dreams in life we must first have a certain amount of desire within us. Ultimately no one can make you do anything. We can be inspired and encouraged but it is our own level of desire that determines whether we take those first steps towards our goals. After that we need determination, perseverance and consistency of effort if we are to realise our ambitions. If we don't maintain our motivation, usually we will find the task too taxing to complete and give up too soon. Motivation often wanes, especially if you are trying break through new barriers or reach hoped for goals you may be a little doubtful of achieving. You need constant reminders of why you want to achieve a certain thing (use the sections on Goals and Personal Affirmations) and then you need to keep up your own confidence by reminding yourself that you are indeed capable of completing the task (use the sections on Affirmations and Positive Thinking). The seed of desire must be within you in the first place. If you really cannot do something that is within your power to achieve then you have to ask yourself what your true intentions are. If you really want something you will achieve it. Where there is a will there is always a way.

 Here are some examples of ways to stay motivated and inspired, tools to keep you going when the going gets a little tough:

- Music can inspire, excite and relax. Choose something that is uplifting to listen to before, during and after you go to meet your challenges.

- Use your personal affirmations to keep up your self-belief and confidence (see Chapter 5)

- Motivational books and audio tapes, videos and DVDs.

- Visual aids. Use magazines or photos of images that show the goals that you are striving to reach, i.e. healthy body, new home, car, etc.

- Maintain fresh goals. We all need something to aim for and work towards.

- Mentors are all around. Start socialising with the type of people you feel are successful with goals similar to your own. Ask them what kept them going. Look for inspiration. Share ideas and thoughts.

- Action and accomplishment. Nothing motivates a person more than being appreciated for doing something good and right. The first steps may be the toughest but things really get rolling when you start producing. However small the progress it is so valuable when you prove to yourself that you can get things done!

- Sometimes past disappointments can spur you on to new accomplishments. Don't let past failure get you down and discourage you. Try again, be better prepared and determined to succeed. Don't wait until you feel your motivation is on its way out! Use these things hourly, daily or as often as possible.

MENTAL TOUGHNESS

It is so important to have some kind of mental toughness. You hear about it all the time in sports and business but every day life tests your ability to be brave and overcome adversity. We all have our challenges and difficulties and it is how we react to these that goes a long way to determining our ability to survive and prosper. That is why we must try not to resent adversity but see it as an opportunity to grow and learn in some way. We are never given more than we can actually take, so we have to learn to deal with what is in front of us and learn from our experiences. If they are recurring problems then it should become clear that this is something that we haven't addressed yet. At the same time as accepting and appreciating our challenges and lessons, it is important to continue to do the things that develop our physical fitness and mental toughness so that we are more able to cope with the stresses and strains of life.

Just as in sport and military service, people are trained to be physically and mentally tough. We too need to do at least some of this, otherwise we, more often than not, find life a little too tough. This is why it is important to set ourselves challenging yet attainable goals and make sure we accomplish them. Remember, the mind is just like a muscle and needs regular training and testing otherwise we get soft and tend to give in easily when under pressure. A lot of mental toughness is about seeing something through to its conclusion, not flunking out when the going gets a bit rough or things become uncomfortable. One of the biggest differences between people who have successfully achieved their goals and dreams and those who fall short is their added mental strength, their determination to push through, the self-belief that keeps them going and the appreciation that there will be difficulties along the way.

You can easily be one of those people. You have just as much of a chance, you just have to decide how much you are willing to put in. You must really care and try to do the best you can, anything less will make it so much easier to fail and not complete the course. Those wonderful feelings of accomplishment and progress that we crave to boost our self-confidence and personal powers do not come cheap. Great relationships are not always love and roses as are successful businesses or creative endeavours. There is always adversity to deal and with you'd better be tough and determined if you want to get what you want and need out of life. The more you take the easy option the harder it is to overcome adversity when it does come, and it will. So relish the tough times as well as the easy times. These are gifts for you too; you just have to recognise that they are there to make you stronger as you rise to the challenge. The stronger you are the easier life gets. After all it is still survival of the fittest. Nothing really has changed in this regard.

GOAL SETTING

Courage is like a muscle, we strengthen it with use

Ruth Gordon

If you don't know where you're going, how will you get there? Setting goals is certainly an important ingredient of life. Goals give us an extra reason to get up in the morning. They focus, motivate and sustain us. Many of us today are just existing because we have given upon our goals. Maybe you have tried and failed to achieve certain things and after a while have resigned yourself to defeat and settled for a lesser life. Maybe you have been the kind of person who has always been afraid to really go for what you want or even stopped completely trying to achieve something more for yourself for various reasons. Maybe you don't know what it is that you want and therefore don't have any goals or aims to work towards. A life without goals is a journey with no destination. Imagine getting into your car, driving off and realising you don't know where you are headed. It's easy to get lost, frustrated and disheartened with no target or destination. Not only do we need goals to keep us motivated and focused, we need the achievement that goes with reaching them to feel like we are making that all important progress in life; we get a kick out of accomplishing something and the sense that we are better off somehow for it. Goals give us this and more. They keep our minds on the prize. They define what we want. They guide our way and set our targets. If you really want change in your life and if you want to make more things happen for yourself and those around you, this is an extremely important part of the programme for you. Try not to think of all this as being too self-centred. The better you are, the more you accomplish and improve, the happier and more fulfilled you are, the more everyone around you benefits.

Dare to Dream

If you know your ultimate goals and dreams then write them in the space provided in Long Term Goals All the important aspects of life are covered and these will help you formulate your various objectives. Please do not pull any punches when you detail what it is you really want. If your intent is good, you wish it with all your heart and you believe it would be genuinely good for you, then write each one down. With belief and perseverance, a lot of hard work and a little luck, there is no reason why you should not attain them. If you do not know what you want, then don't worry, just follow this programme and work on developing yourself. Aim to get healthy and back in touch with yourself. Soon your mind will become uncluttered and the road ahead will become clear.

Any medium or long term goals require short term goals as stepping stones. It is vitally important if you want to reach your larger and more distant goals to maintain your focus and productivity with daily and weekly goals and 'To Do's'. In the section on Time Management, I suggest that you get yourself a time management tool like a planner or diary to help you stay organised. These all should have a To Do section and you would do well to keep up with your immediate obligations and targets if you are going to stay the course. Set goals for all the major aspects of your life – career, financial, fitness and physique, family, organisation, education and hobbies. Sometimes your goals change which is why there are repeat pages for you to develop your ideas and update you goals and dreams. Keep wishing, keep dreaming, keep working and keep achieving. You WILL get there.

Life Aspect	Goals
Physical	....
	....
	....
	....
Career	....
	....
	....
	....
Family	....
	....
	....
	....
Lifestyle	....
	....
	....
	....
Personal	....
	....
	....
	....

Write down your long term, life goals, dreams and wishes here. Imagine them coming true. Make sure it is a win/win for all and have the best intentions behind them. See the section on the Creative Process to learn more effectively how to harness your creative powers as you work towards these.

Life Aspect	Goals
Physical	....
	....
	....
	....
Career	....
	....
	....
	....
Family	....
	....
	....
	....
Lifestyle	....
	....
	....
	....
Personal	....
	....
	....
	....

Write down the mid term (roughly two to four months) goals here. These are helpful targets.

TIME MANAGEMENT

No man can paddle two canoes at the same time

Bantu Proverb

Your time, along with your health, is probably your most valuable asset. This is your life and how you apportion your time determines your present and your future situation. Time is money and the efficient use of it will determine whether you have the freedom to do what you want, or stay trapped in a cycle of obligation and working for others. You may already be finding that your time is being completely consumed in this way, or you may be taking time out to reassess your goals, career and desired schedule. Whatever position you are in, if you want to be healthy and fulfilled, you must maintain a basic balance to your time expenditure. Be organised and efficient, value and protect your free time and, above all, make sure you get your basic needs met every day as a matter of course. Here are some helpful tips concerning time management and being better organised.

- Scheduling your time really begins with work for most people, so being organised starts with using tools to stay organised and efficient. There are some very useful time management systems on the market that you would be wise to use. A planner, whether electronic or the binder variety, allows you not only to plan your obligations but also track your time expenditure in a log. This enables you to see how much time you are spending in certain tasks, so enabling you to adjust as needed.

- Planners usually encompass comprehensive To Do lists. It is important to fill these out when the task arises and keep them up-to-date as tasks are executed. Your To Do's have an order of importance so you will want to prioritise your lists as you go.

- Being organised saves you a lot of time, so spending a certain amount of time a day making sure all your affairs are in order saves time in the long run.

- Keeping your paperwork tidy and filing things away neatly helps a lot too. Avoid having hundreds of pieces of paper and business cards hanging around. Log any new contacts in your diary or phone book every day and transfer information into your main organiser whenever you get it. If you do a little organisation each day you will soon get into the habit.

- Understand what you can realistically achieve with your time. Start by identifying the time you want to make available for your work. This will depend on the design of your job and on your personal goals.

- Next, block in the actions you absolutely must take to do a good job. These will help you work more efficiently by doing things right the first time. For example, if you manage people, then you must make time for dealing with issues that arise, coaching and supervision. Similarly, you must allow time to communicate with your boss and key people around you. While people may let you get away with neglecting them in the short term, your best time management efforts will surely be derailed if you do not set aside time for the important people in your life.

- Review your To Do list and schedule in the high priority urgent activities, as well as the essential maintenance tasks that cannot be delegated or avoided.

- Block in appropriate contingency time. You will learn how much of this you need from experience. Normally, the more unpredictable your job, the more contingency time you need. The reality of many people's work is one of constant interruption. Obviously, you cannot anticipate when they will occur but, by leaving space in your schedule, you give yourself the flexibility to react effectively to issues as they arise.

- What you now have left is your 'discretionary time': the time available to deliver your priorities and achieve your goals. Review your Prioritised To Do List and Personal Goals and evaluate the time needed to achieve these actions, and schedule these in.

YOUR HEALTH PRIORITIES

To maintain a healthy body and mind, and avoid excessive stress build up, we have to find time each day for three nutritious meals, plenty of water intake, exercise and stretching (even just a little before bed is good and very important), positive thinking and goal setting, reflection, relaxation, preparation for the next day and seven to nine hours of good and restful sleep. If each day contains these elements you will be giving yourself the best chance of coping with any stress and be alert enough to take advantage of opportunities as they arise. So can you get into this healthy habit on work and weekend days, busy times and not so busy times? Whether young or old, we all need these basics in our lives and until we get into the habit of including them, we will always find life a little more difficult than we should. It may seem like a lot but it's really not too much to ask of yourself. These really are the basic and simplest requirements for your wellbeing to give you a good work/life balance.

This is a list that truly intelligent people follow because it is a routine that ensures you get your basic needs met. Remember, true intelligence is expressed by knowing what you are, doing what you do and getting what you need. Plants and animals do this instinctively. We need to be reminded. The world and our busy schedules distract us from really applying our intelligence, being ourselves and living according to our nature. We all have obligations but our main one is to ourselves. Our health underpins any prosperity that we might enjoy so it is time to figure out our priorities as we create a new lifestyle. If you are sacrificing your wellbeing for perceived personal gain and success, those achievements will be short lived. Be organised, be prepared, be balanced and above all, be happy!

1. **On waking, remember your goals and repeat your affirmations. Give yourself enough time for breakfast and to prepare for the day. Take 20 extra minutes, you will need it (see Affirmations section)**

2. **Drink some fresh water (we all wake up dehydrated, so drink!)**

3. **Eat a nutritious breakfast (take plenty of time, try not to rush into your day).**

4. **Drink a glass of water per hour during the day.**

5. **Eat a nutritious lunch (sit down and eat).**

6. **Try to stretch and exercise after work or school as part of the buffer between your work and private time.**

7. **Read a little to calm and slow down your mind.**

8. **Repeat your affirmations and count your blessings each day.**

9. **Plan the next day the evening before using your planner and complete your next To Do list.**

10. **Set boundaries with your work so that you have time to relax and enjoy a little personal and family down time in the evening. Learn to say no and defend your free time.**

11. **It is so important mentally and emotionally to let the day go and get ready for a good restful sleep. Don't eat too late and don't let the business of the day continue into the night. Practice releasing and use your affirmations to help you (see Chapter 5).**

MENU PLANNER

As this is the part of the book that is encouraging you to be organised and maintain your work/life balance, I felt it appropriate to place the menu and activity planner here. You may want to read the upcoming sections on healthy eating and exercise first and when you have, you can return to complete these planners. Remember this book is all about being your best. We all need to work hard to achieve our goals but it is vital to maintain our energy daily if we are going to stay the course. Use this menu planner and design a couple of different days' eating depending on whether it is a work day or off day and allow for some variety. Your eating is your most important physical need so this may be the most important part of this plan.

You are about to learn all you need to know about eating. It is so important that you plan your healthy eating day. Plan your own daily and weekly menus on the following pages.

Date:

Breakfast

....

....

....

....

Lunch

....

....

....

....

Snack

....

....

....

....

Dinner

....

....

....

....

Date:

Breakfast

....

....

....

....

Lunch

....

....

....

....

Snack

....

....

....

....

Dinner

....

....

....

....

Date:

Breakfast

....

....

....

....

Lunch

....

....

....

....

Snack

....

....

....

....

Dinner

....

....

....

....

ACTIVITY PLANNER

Use this space to plan a typical week of exercise and activity. It is part of your preparation and time management to decide what activity you intend to do on which particular day, depending on your schedule, obligations, options and your need for rest. If you are not the kind of person who finds it easy to exercise and do sports, then this is especially important for you. This plan should reflect the goals you have set for yourself concerning your fitness and physique, and show your intention for necessary lifestyle change. Get off the couch or away from your computer and go and do something healthy for yourself. When you know you have particularly stressful days and really need to get out and blow the cobwebs off, then schedule activity accordingly. When you are particularly busy, plan something quick and easy to do like a brief yoga routine or a little dancing to music at home. Try to plan something every day that gets your heart rate up and gives you a good stretch. You will enjoy it and before you know it, it will become habit.

Monday..

....

....

....

....

Tuesday..

....

....

....

Wednesday..

....

....

....

Thursday ....

....

....

....

....

Friday ....

....

....

....

....

Saturday..

....

....

....

....

Sunday...

....

....

....

....

CHAPTER FOUR

Getting Stronger

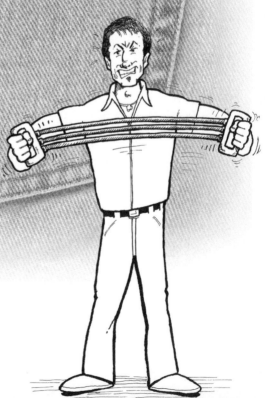

YOUR PHYSICAL POTENTIAL

If we don't take care of our body, where will we live?

Proverb

We all inhabit a body in this life. We may not like it, but we must learn to love it and appreciate it if we are going to live a long, energetic and fulfilling life. Few of us realise our true physical potential. Granted, not many of us actually want to put ourselves through what we perceive to be significant pain and discomfort to reach our physical peak. The problem is, many of us hate the prospect of exercise and healthy eating so much that we are not prepared to put up with any discomfort or pain to realise better health and consequent quality of life. Therefore we make do with feeling tired, overweight, stiff and less attractive even though this ultimately makes us unhappy. We may hate the fact, but we have to care for our bodies if we want to feel and look half decent.

Today, where machines do much of our strenuous work for us, we have forgotten what stimulation, nutrition and training our body still needs if it is going to operate properly and maintain our basic physical integrity. Our bodies are incredibly adept at self regulation and equilibrium. Just like the most advanced machines, our muscles, joints, internal organs, circulatory and immune systems as well as our brains, need to be serviced and tested regularly as well as fed with a constant and quality supply of energy and fresh air. Otherwise the body just breaks down prematurely. Bodies can turn ugly in a hurry when we mistreat them.

We can't keep ignoring their needs and expect them just to keep going no matter what we put them through. The energy we expend, our appearance and performance, is wholly related to the quality of energy and care that goes into our systems. We are an energy transformer. We take it in and we put it out. We have amazing potential for output that few realise and appreciate fully. It isn't necessary to go to extremes to discover our potential. We just need to give our bodies, as well as our minds and inner selves (as all are connected), what they require and use them for whatever we want to do. Instead of accepting poor energy, looks and performance because we can't be bothered to invest the care and attention that we need for our physical wellbeing, maybe it is time to educate ourselves and remember what these beautiful and near perfect organic 'machines' are capable of and what they need to function optimally.

Our body's top ten needs are:

1. **Oxygen** – Oxygen heals and revitalises the body and mind. Physical and breathing exercises are required regularly.

2. **Water** – You need a minimum of eight glasses per day.

3. **Nutrition** – Three nutritious meals and a snack per day.

4. **Sleep** – Seven to nine hours, depending on your body. Relaxation and stretching before bed helps restful sleep.

5 **Exercise** – It's more than necessary for maintenance of physical abilities and energy flow; it's a celebration of being fit and alive!

6. **Stretching** – Good health depends on good posture and being free of muscular tension.

7. **Hygiene** – Keep yourself and your environment clean for good health.

8. **Touch/Hugs/Massage** – It's all good. Make it loving and fun!

9. **Communication** – Listen to your body. It knows when something is wrong and listens to the messages you send to it.

10. **Relaxation** – Become a relaxed person by taking time to relax every day. Laugh, be entertained, be quiet, be passive and be still, even if only for a few minutes. It is part of your vital balance.

Don't underestimate the wisdom of your body. Get better at listening to it and make sure you are positive about it and appreciate it as much as you can. In addition to these needs, we also require regular:

• **Sunlight** – Sunshine has amazing healing qualities and benefits.

• **Resistance** – Our bodies need resistance to stay strong.

- **Movement** – We must move our bodies to maintain our range of motion and to celebrate the fact that we can.

- **Massage** – Keeps muscles toned and circulation sound. Improves and maintains mind/body connection and satisfies our need for touch too.

- **Laughter** – Apart from emptying the lungs of old, stale air, it provides life prolonging and vitality stimulating hormones, as well as toning muscles and letting off steam.

- **Pain** – Vital feedback. It tells us when something is wrong.

- **Grooming** – Got to look like we know how to look after ourselves, after all, we live in a 'first impression' world.

- **Rhythm** – There is a time for everything, try to maintain a rhythm in your life, sleeping, eating, working, etc.

- **Music** – Stimulates the body and relieves tension.

- **Tools** – Can't do a proper job without the right tools.

- **Training** – There is a right way to do everything. Our bodies respond well to training. Learn how to do things right, be accomplished and save a lot of time.

- **Time** – Use it well and don't rush things.

- **Protection** – Stay safe, be protected.

- **Space** – We all need to feel we have enough space to live and breathe freely. Respect yours and other people's.

- **Intimacy** – A little bit of love goes a long way.

- **Quiet** – In a world with so much noise, quiet can be just what you need sometimes. Make time for it. What are you missing and how is your body suffering because of this lack?

We are now going to cover the main needs in a little more depth.

BETTER EATING AND SHOPPING FOR THE GOOD STUFF

 You eat crap and you'll look and feel like crap too! Sorry, harsh but true. Good nutrition is the most fundamental need of your body.

The main goal of good nutrition is to supply all the elements the body needs for correct functioning. We are in a constant need for refueling and repair. If you want to look good and feel good you need to eat right. Everything you eat has a profound and lasting effect on your whole self, not just your body. Your brainpower, your moods, your energy levels and basic physical appearance are directly related to what you eat. You really are what you eat. If you eat highly processed fast food you are not getting the nutrients you need to fuel and repair your body and you will also be taking in dangerous amounts of salt, saturated fat and chemicals. If you are active, you need to take extra care to get the nutrients you need.

We are digging our graves with our teeth

Samuel Pepys

Let's learn a bit more about food. Food is divided into three main components. These are protein, fat and carbohydrate. Each component is unique and necessary to the body and each one has different effects and provides different individual nutrients. Balancing them is very important. Food can be a very powerful drug. Unless taken in balanced form, moderate quantity and nutritious quality, it can have many undesirable effects. Countless studies prove that if we ate whole, unprocessed and nutritionally satisfying food, we would not suffer nearly as many sicknesses as we do and we wouldn't need all the drugs and remedies so many of us

52

take. If you have become run down and sick you really can heal yourself with good food. It is as simple as that. Food is our greatest medicine. In addition to supplying the body with nutrients, the other goal of sensible eating is to keep a steady energy supply. When your blood sugar is stable, your energy will be good, your moods balanced and your appetite in check.

When you eat balanced and nutritionally healthy food you will feel satisfied after each meal and have lasting and steady energy leaving you ready to be productive. When you eat poorly balanced meals, high in fat, salt or processed carbohydrates and sugars, your blood sugar will be unstable and you will experience quite the opposite. You feel irritable – craving sweets – and lethargic and this, in turn, makes it almost impossible to eat healthily and maintain weight. To keep blood sugar steady, you must always try to eat your meals with the correct balance of protein, fat and carbohydrate. Many of the body's systems rely on this balance and the entire organism is thrown out when food is eaten in the wrong proportions. It simply means that the body does much better when meals have equal calories coming from protein, fat and carbohydrate sources. This may not be the ratio you have seen before but I have found that it's the easiest to manage and it creates a steady blood sugar level to provide maximum energy. Remember though that each group has a different calorie content so you will have to eat less fat than protein and plenty more green vegetable carbohydrates as they contain fewer calories per gram than the others.

 Remember: Fat has twice as many calories per gram than protein and carbohydrates so adjust accordingly in your portions.

- Carbohydrates: Starchy veggies (e.g. potatoes, corn, lima beans, sweet potatoes), pasta, rice, alcohol, bread, cakes, cookies, sweets, fruits. (Salads and green vegetables are slightly different as they have much fewer calories and generally more fibre than these other carbs so you can eat a greater quantity of these.)

- Proteins: Meat, seafood, tofu, soy protein, milk, eggs, beans, spinach, protein powders. Not only is oily fish is a great source of protein but it is also extremely effective in improving concentration and is calming to the mind.

- Fats: Oils, avocados, cheese (has protein and carbs also), nuts, seeds, butter, mayonnaise, margarine, cream.

For steady blood sugar and body balance, it is also important to eat meals at regular intervals. Do not skip meals. Make good healthy natural choices when selecting from your three main components. You also need to know how important it is that you do not eat these components on their own, only within properly balanced and complete meals. Avoid adding extra salt to meals.

Recap:

- **Eat balanced meals at meal times.**

- **Eat small portions.**

- **Eat meals with fresh food as often as possible. Avoid fast, processed food.**

- **Especially avoid eating carbohydrates on their own.**

- **TAKE TIME TO PREPARE AND ENJOY YOUR FOOD. YOU GET OUT WHAT YOU PUT IN!**

It is important to note that some choices are better than others of the three main nutritional components. An obvious example when choosing protein foods is to select good free range, hormone and antibiotic free, lean meats rather than fattier, processed meats. The same goes for carbohydrates. We have talked a lot about whole foods and this is especially important when choosing your carbs. Whole grain breads, rice and pasta are much better than the whiter variety. Also fruits that have more fibre like berries, apples, pears and pineapple make better choices. If you are trying to lose fat, then avoid starchy carbs like pasta, bread and potatoes in favour of green veggies and salads. Oils and fats need to come from natural foods like seeds, avocados, oily fish, nuts and even a little real butter is good for you. Avoid fats from fried food or refined vegetable oils. Good fats transport vitamins so you really do need good fat in your diet. Choose wisely.

DRINKING HABITS

You probably know that too much alcohol can damage the liver but other parts of the body, including the heart, can also be harmed if you drink excessively on a regular basis. Remember that more than 21 units of alcohol for a man and 14 units for a woman can damage health. If you drink more than 49 units per week there is a definite risk of developing serious problems. (A unit is the equivalent of one glass of wine or beer or a shot of spirits). If you want to maintain your health and your weight, it is better to consume alcoholic drinks with meals. These drinks are predominantly carbohydrates which will cause blood sugar spikes and weight gain, especially around the waist. If you want to drink but still maintain your weight, then eat less carbohydrates with meals.

Important Points

Quantity: If you picture a regular dinner plate, a regular, sensible meal should fill it (not piled up). The protein should make up a third of the plate, the carbs another third and vegetables or salad the last third. This type of meal will give you the nutrients you need as long as ingredients are whole and fresh. There are a number of factors in which you contribute to quantity control:

1. **Stay organised**. Plan your meals the night before. Know where you are going to be and plan what you are going to eat. Be prepared.

2. **Start the day off right**. A balanced breakfast sets the tone for the day keeping blood sugar and appetite in check for the day.

3. **Meal spacing**. Eating full balanced meals no less than three hours and no more than five hours apart will ensure steady energy and appetite control which will determine quantity at each meal especially dinner. Have a healthy snack at hand if there is a big gap between your meals.

4. **Fibre**. If you eat foods rich in fibre, they tend to fill you up and be more satisfying than foods that have little fibre. Remember foods with fibre are always carbohydrates and need to be part of a meal with protein and fats as well. Fibre is found in bran cereals, whole grain bread, green vegetables and other fruits (not bananas), beans and lentils, etc.

5. **Drink water with meals**. You need eight full glasses of water a day. Drink one with each meal. It will make sure you fill up and are satisfied.

6. **Eating out**. Most dishes in sauces are high in fat, salt and sugar. To ensure you maintain your healthy eating programme avoid sauces and eat your proteins grilled or stir-fried. In restaurants be sure to ask that the dish be kept as free from fat, salt and sugar as possible.

7. **Treats**. It is important that you do not make your diet too strict. Give yourself a treat regularly, in fact, factor it in to your eating plan, e.g. eat what you want one day per week but try not to go too crazy. Remember this is a reward not self-abuse.

8. **Comfort eating.** Make sure you deal with stress effectively and be organised. When you are overwhelmed, depressed or stressed out you tend to make poor choices and overeat. Avoid highly processed food filled with fat, salt and preservatives.

Portions and Proportions: Remembering the philosophy of balance, there should not be any portion of protein or carbohydrate on your plate larger than will fit in the palm of your hand (no more than 6 oz or 160 grams). Carbohydrate foods should also fit in your hand. No more than 1 cup (what will fit in a normal cup) cooked or ½ cup uncooked for starches such as pasta, rice or potatoes. Veggies can be eaten in large quantities (less for carrots). Bread (choose whole grain variety) and no more than two slices each meal with equal amounts of meat or protein.

Remember: Balance Always! This is the most simple and sensible way to eat.

EATING FOR PERFORMANCE

To maintain performance during long periods of activity or exercise make sure you take in small amounts of balanced, unprocessed and fresh food regularly. This should have some protein in it too. Egg sandwiches, protein bars, trail mix, peanut butter on crackers and fruit are some good choices.

SHOPPING

Just look through the Meal and Snacks and your meal planner sections to know what you need to shop for. Typically, you are always going to need meats, fish, eggs, nuts, salads, bread, dairy, vegetables and fruit. The items are usually found around the perimeter of the grocery store. If you find yourself going down the isles for food, ask yourself if you really need it? Do you have a meal to put it in which will have the essential balance of protein, fat and carbohydrate for the body? Try to buy more fruit and vegetables instead of cereals, bread, potatoes and pasta when planning meals. Again, look at options and plan accordingly.

Recap:

- **Shop more around the perimeter of the store**
- **Shop regularly for fresh food**
- **Don't shop hungry!**
- **Remember you will eat what you buy!**
- **Park far away and walk to store**
- **Make shopping exercise**
- **Think ahead to your future schedules**
- **Be prepared!**

Eating healthily begins with good and regular shopping. Here is a sample of a shopping list that reminds you of all the necessary aspects of a good diet that you need to have in your home. Keep this as a template.

Shopping list

Write out a sample list and get into the habit of buying in good food and being prepared. Some examples to get you started.

Type of Food	Variety	Where From
PROTEIN	Tofu, turkey breast, eggs, cheese	Grocery store
CARBS	Rice, oatmeal etc	Health food store
VEGGIES/SALADS		
FRUITS		
SNACKS		
WATER		
DRINKS		
SUPPLEMENTS		

GOOD MEAL CHOICES

These are some examples of good, healthy and balanced meals.

Breakfasts

1. 3 egg omelette (1 yolk), cheese and veggies, 1 piece toast and jam, glass natural juice

2. 2 poached eggs on wholewheat toast with juice

3. Cottage cheese and fruit

4. Natural yoghurt and nuts

5. Scrambled egg and sausage wrap (scrambled eggs, meat free sausage, low fat cheese and salsa), glass of juice

6. Toasted egg and bacon sandwich (I egg and 2 slices bacon, fry in small amount of oil, 2 slices wholewheat bread)

7. Cereals. Note: when you eat cereal make sure you have small portions, be aware of the sugar content and eat protein with it.
I cup of low sugar, low fat Shredded Wheat, All Bran, Muesli, Special K, Bran Flakes, Whole grain Cheerios with one cup of low fat milk and a handful nuts

Lunches

1. Chef salad (1/2 bag tossed salad, 1 egg, ½ cup crumbled feta cheese, onion, pepper, cucumber, etc, oil and vinegar, fruit or yogurt). Add protein choice for balance

2. Can of low fat soup, 2 hard-boiled eggs, piece of fruit. Note: when purchasing soup, watch for sodium content and fat

3. Sandwiches. Any high fibre bread with salads, vegetables and protein. Make sure there is balance here and a sandwich can be a healthy meal in itself. Add piece of fruit or yoghurt for extra vitamins and protein

4. Tuna pita pocket with salad and veggies. Tuna or chicken pasta or rice salad

5. Baked potato with tuna, beans and cheese or just with cottage cheese and salad for fewer calories

6. High protein fruit smoothie

7. Smoked mackerel salad and new potatoes

Chinese

1. Chicken with snow peas and small rice

2. Chicken with mixed vegetables

3. Prawns with broccoli and rice

4. Beef with snow peas and small rice

Dinner

1. Chicken breast (grilled) with rice and veggies

2. Baked potato, cottage cheese, tuna and salad

3. Chicken breast sandwich with fruit

4. Corned beef sandwich or grilled ham with pineapple

5. Hamburger patty or cottage cheese, salad and fruit

6. Pork chop, baked potato and vegetables

7. Baked fish with small rice or potato and veggies

8. Grilled chicken salad and fruit

9. Meat or seafood stir fry

Take a little time to learn a few new recipes and get into cooking. This can be relaxing as well as tremendously good for your overall health. When you shop well and cook at home, you know what is going into your food. Be adventurous, keep the ingredients of high quality, and enjoy your food. You are not only what you eat but how you eat.

Snacks

Trail Mix (nuts, seeds and dried fruit)

Peanut butter crackers

Power or Balance bar

Yoghurt with nuts

Soy nuts and piece of fruit

EVALUATE YOUR CURRENT EATING

Take a week or so to evaluate what you are putting in your body at the moment. Use the evaluation charts over the next few pages. Be honest. Sometimes it can only get better.

Breakfast

....

....

....

Lunch

....

....

....

Snack

....

....

....

Dinner

....

....

....

Date:

Comments:

....

....

Breakfast

....
....
....

Lunch

....
....
....

Snack

....
....
....

Dinner

....
....
....

Date:

Comments:

....
....

Breakfast

....
....
....

Lunch

....
....
....

Snack

....
....
....

Dinner

....
....
....

Date:

Comments:

....
....

Breakfast

....
....
....

Lunch

....
....
....

Snack

....
....
....

Dinner

....
....
....

Date:

Comments:

....
....

GETTING FITTER

Clothes put on while running come off while running

Ethiopian Proverb

So you want to look great, feel great and have plenty of energy, right? You want to be less stressed, better able to cope with the challenges of life and be more successful? Then you've got to exercise. Exercise is fun and quick if done right. Plus it kind of gets addictive after a while so, once you get into exercise, it's hard to stop. Man has known for centuries about the effect exercise has on the body and mind, but we seem to forget sometimes. If you are not exercising, you are probably making do with an inferior quality of life that you need to change. You need to raise your standards and expectations for yourself (see section on Motivation). Getting exercise is easy when you make the commitment to health and wellbeing; give yourself a wide choice and find something you like. The choices given here in this section make it easy and fun to choose what particular exercise and activity you want to do each day and really enjoy it. That's what sports, dance and athletics were invented for. It's exercise made fun. It's also a challenge.

Exercise (as well as healthy eating) is the greatest weapon against ageing and sickness we know today! Exercise stimulates vital hormones, which deteriorate when we get older or are sick. These hormones keep us strong, sharp and vital. If you love life, you should love to exercise. But if you don't, it's not that difficult to get going. Exercising will remind you how great life can be. It is also a basic need. If you briefly look back at the 'Puzzle of Life', you will see quite a few needs that can be incorporated just by starting to exercise.

 Remember the golden rule: Take care of YOUR health first. EVERYONE around you benefits.

Exercise a Little and Make the World of Difference

Our bodies need resistance, stretching, regular postural alignment and regular aerobic activity to be fit for life. You don't need that much, just something regularly. The strength and stretching bit follows shortly but let's start with the most important, the aerobic part. Aerobics literally means 'with oxygen' and such exercise places emphasis on maintaining a consistent heart rate over an extended period of time. Cardiovascular fitness represents the body's ability to take in oxygen and distribute it to the muscles and other parts of the body, including the brain. The heart and lungs are the core of the cardiovascular system. When your cardiovascular fitness improves, you will have more energy throughout the day and will increase overall endurance. Aerobic exercise causes the heart to pump harder, but should not make you short of breath. Take extra time to warm up before exercise and cool down after your workout. Also, check with your physician before beginning an exercise programme.

Aerobic Activity

In order to achieve your fitness goal, you need to do something aerobic at least every other day: start with 15 minutes of aerobic activity and work up to 30–45 minutes if you can. To maximise your time spent doing aerobic activity, you need to be exercising within your target heart rate zone. It doesn't matter what you choose to do as long as it gets your heart rate up for a sustained period of time, makes you sweat and breathe hard as a result and hopefully is something you enjoy. Here are some examples:

1. Swimming
2. Cycling
3. Dancing
4. Gardening
5. Running/Jogging
6. Aerobics Class
7. Active Sports
8. Active Sex
9. Gym Workout
10. Power Walking

Keep it fun and challenging but don't overdo it. Try to look forward to your exercises and see it as a celebration of your body and life. Feel lucky that you can do these things at all. (See section on positive thinking and affirmations.)

Aerobic Activity and Fat Loss

If it is your intention to lose body fat, the aerobic activity will speed up the process. When the heart is worked at a steady rate in the 65–75% (not above) then the energy used for this activity comes almost exclusively from fat. If, however, as with weight training or more strenuous activity, the heart rate is taken above 80%, then more and more energy comes from the glycogen (stored sugars) inside the muscle. Regardless of whether it is morning or evening, doing it any time is better than not doing it at all. After you have finished and are warm and sweaty this would be a good time to do your stretching routine which you need for all around fitness and wellbeing (see next section).

Warming Up and Cooling Down

Whenever you plan to do any strenuous physical activity or sport, it is very important to warm up and cool down properly. It is so easy to injure yourself if you are not warmed up and stretched. Preparation is everything. For muscles and joints to be fully prepared to perform at their best, they need some basic stretching and warm up exercises. You don't need a full cardio and stretch workout to get ready for action. A small amount of jogging, cycling and star jumps will do the job of general warming up and a few simple stretches shown below will get the muscles and joints ready to go. After activity, especially if it has been particularly challenging, you must cool down and stretch in the same way or the muscles will tighten and knot up. Shorter muscles and tight joints are very vulnerable to injury, premature fatigue, pain and discomfort. Take the time to do this and you will always be ready to do your best!

Warm Up and Cool Down Routine

After a brief warm up these movements and stretches will help you prepare for your activity, whatever it is. Turn to the stretching section and perform movements 3 to13.These exercises will prepare your body and also focus your mind. A gentle jog and a repeat of recommended stretches plus the corpse pose (No.20) will provide you with the right kind of cool down after your session. If you are playing in a sports competition and have to wait between rounds or matches you must still warm up and cool down each time. Remember; it only takes 10 minutes or so to do these exercises but it takes many weeks to get over injuries.

Target Heart Rate Zones

Ages	Beats/10 Seconds
18	20–29
19–25	20–28
26–32	9–27
33–35	19–26
36–40	18–25
41–47	17–25
48–54	17–24
55	17–23
56–61	16–23
62–65	16–22
66–68	15–22
69–70	15–21

How to Check Heart Rate and What it Means:

As you can see, the above shows the sensible heart rate ranges which you should try to maintain during your cardiovascular workout whatever it is you are doing: dancing, walking, swimming, jogging, stair climbing (all these are good aerobic exercises). Begin slowly and increase your pace gradually. Be sure to check your heart rate until you reach your required zone. This could take 5–10 minutes. When you reach it, try to maintain the time dictated by your programme depending on experience or fitness levels. To check your heart rate, place index finger and middle finger on your wrist (near base of thumb, side of wrist) or neck slightly below your ear. When you find your pulse count the beats for ten seconds and multiply by six and you have your beats per minute. A heart rate monitor would be a great investment to make sure of efficiency of effort. The best time of the day to do fat loss aerobics is first thing in the morning before breakfast because the body is already in a state of fasting, there is no food in the stomach and this ensures a good climate for fat loss. After work is also a good time as it gives you chance to burn off any extra calories you may have 'accidentally' taken in during the day. It is also a great stress reliever.

STRETCHING AWAY THE STRESS: OVERCOMING TENSION AND AVOIDING POWER LOSS

 You got to loosen up, dude.

Tension is one of the major causes of aches and pains, poor sleep and bad posture and it even compounds psychological problems such as anger, frustration, anxiety and impatience. Life can make us so tense at times. When we get stressed and lose our tempers, when we slouch or sit in bad positions, when we use our muscles repetitively and don't stretch out at the end of each day, we accumulate tension and it gradually gets worse. When we go to bed with this tension, which we don't necessarily release during sleep, our quality of sleep suffers and we often wake up the next day still full of tension and often tired and irritable from the previous day.

He who has health has hope, and he who has hope has everything

Saudi Arabian Proverb

Top Ten Reasons to Stretch Every Day

1. Reduces muscle tension and make the body feel more relaxed.

2. Helps coordination allowing for freer and easier movement.

3. Improves posture.

4. Increases range of motion.

5. Helps prevent injuries such as muscle strains when done before and after physical activity.

6. Develops body awareness. As you stretch various parts of the body, you focus on them and get feedback from them.

7. Promotes good circulation which is vital for your overall health and ability to fight off disease.

8. Speeds muscle recovery.

9. It slows down the brain, relieves stress and feels good.

10. Tones muscles, increases metabolism and makes it easy to maintain a lean body.

The Stretches

Important points about stretching:

*   Take slow deep breaths. Try to exhale as you begin to move into the stretched positions. When you feel tension or pressure, do not hold your breath. Do not stretch to the point of pain.

*   Never force a stretch. Do not bounce. It takes time for your muscles to get the message to relax. Be patient.

*   It is easier to stretch a warm muscle than a cold one. Whenever possible, try to stretch when you are warmed up from cardiovascular activity (i.e. walking, running, biking or swimming). You can also stretch more easily after training with weights or with resistance bands or even after a warm bath or shower.

*   Use visualisation to help your body feel relaxed and to align yourself properly. Picture your spine being aligned yet flexible and your muscles being lengthened and relaxed. Take a few minutes to meditate on a joyful thought or memory, make it more real with every breath you take. Give yourself positive affirmations (e.g. I am strong, I am happy, I feel fit and flexible, etc.). Your mind is EXTREMELY powerful. Use this power to your advantage. Practice these affirmations daily. Remember if you tell yourself 'I'm stiff', 'I can't stretch, 'I'll never be able to bend' or have any other negative thoughts, your body WILL LISTEN. (See section on positive thinking and affirmations.)

- Be consistent. Try to stretch every day. If time is an issue, stretch the muscles you will be using the most in the upcoming activity or the ones that seem the tightest.

- If you are struggling to reach, grasp or balance while you are stretching, it will be difficult to progress. Try to use the weight of your relaxed body (i.e. relax you head, shoulders, arms, hands, etc.) depending on your position, to help you stretch more deeply. Even clenching your jaw, screwing up your face or tightening your fists can hold you back.

- If you feel any undue stress, strain or pain in the joints, neck or back, be sure to check your position and reread the instructions for the stretch. See your physician if you are unsure about what is safe for you.

The Routine

Before you try any postures, take a moment in a sitting (cross-legged) or prone position (corpse pose) and get in touch with your breath. This is your life force. Inhalations and long exhalations will begin to quiet the mind. You will begin to feel more centred and relaxed. Carry this attitude of focus and balance through your practice and, most importantly, remember to BREATHE. Now let's begin.

1. Mountain Pose

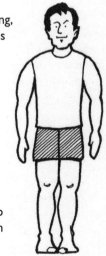

When we think of a mountain, it begins with a strong, broad base. Bring the legs together with the ankles and toes together too, if possible. Think of the feet broadening across the ball of the foot with the toes spreading. Focus on a feeling of drawing upward from the arches of the feet, through the spine, up the back of the neck and through the crown of the head. Keep the chest lifted, shoulders broad with the shoulder blades dropping down your back. Feel a gentle drawing in and lifting up from the lower abdominal area. Let the 'sitting bones' at the bottom of the pelvis draw down so the back does not become swaybacked or alternatively collapsed or slumped. Breathe slow, deep breaths. Count approximately 10 breaths (one inhalation and one exhalation = one breath).

2. Upward Reach

From mountain pose, inhale as you extend the arms over your head, palms facing each other. If bringing the hands together is too uncomfortable for your shoulders then keep the arms shoulder distance apart. Gaze upward towards your fingers, if this is too uncomfortable on your neck then look straight ahead. Keep the shoulders relaxed to avoid any feeling of shrugging. Feel a lifting from underneath the navel area as well as lifting through the sides of the body and from the lower back. Breathe slow deep breaths. Count 5–7 breaths and return to mountain pose.

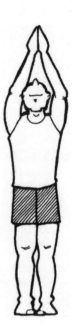

3. Balancing Stick

Look ahead rather than up. Try to keep arms up next to the ears so your head stays between your arms, shoulders relaxed, no shrugging. Step right foot slightly forward, shifting weight on to right leg. Lift left foot off floor and begin to balance forward on right leg. Keep arms in line with raised leg. The body forms a 'T' in the advanced version. Count 5–7 breaths and return to mountain pose. Repeat on opposite side.

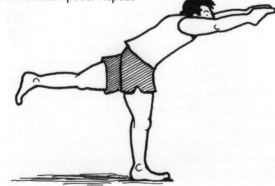

4. Warrior

From mountain pose, extend arms out like aeroplane wings. Step feet apart in wide stance so wrists are in line with sides of feet. Turn toes slightly inward on left foot and on right foot, turn toes fully out to the right (90 degrees). Line up the heel of your right foot with the arch (instep) of your left foot. Turn from your waist so your upper body faces your right leg. Inhale and raise arms above head, palms facing each other and bend your right knee. Continue slow, deep breaths. Do not let the right knee bow in or out to either side. Keep knee in line with the ankle. Shoulders stay back in line over the hips. Left leg (back leg) remains straight. Count 5–7 breaths. Straighten front leg, placing hands on hips. Repeat on opposite side. Good groin stretch.

5. Warrior II

From mountain pose, extend arms out like aeroplane wings, palms facing the floor. Step feet apart in wide stance so wrists are in line with sides of feet. Turn toes slightly inward on left foot and on right foot, turn toes fully out to the right (90 degrees). Line up the heel of your right foot with the arch (instep) of your left foot. Bend your right knee. Do not let the right knee bow in or out to either side. Keep knee in line with the ankle. Keep the shoulders in line with the hips. Left leg (back leg) remains straight. Count 5–7 breaths. Straighten front leg, placing hands on hips. Repeat on opposite side. Stretches hips, buttocks, abdomen and calves.

6. Quad Stretch

For the front of the thighs use a chair to balance, hold foot to buttock as shown and breathe and hold for ten seconds each leg.

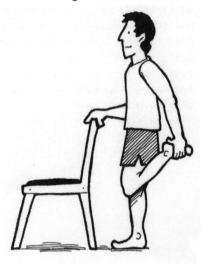

7. Hamstring Stretch

For hamstrings reach for back of chair or wall, keep back and legs straight, lower chest until you feel backs of legs stretching, breathe and hold for ten seconds.

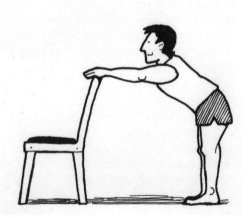

8. Down Dog

Begin in table position and turn your toes under. As you breathe in and exhale, raise up high on the toes coming in a 'V' position. Focus on the hips as you raise them up and back and descend the heels downward. Press the perimeter of the palms of the hands into the mat and feel the energy move out through the fingertips. If your hamstrings are tight, bend the knees slightly to take any rounding of the spine out of the pose. Eventually you will be able to straighten the legs. Allow the head to release and hold the pose while breathing for one minute. This posture not only aligns and elongates the spine, but also builds arm strength. Practise this posture often. It increases blood flow to the brain and has many of the same benefits that headstand does. It also stretches calves and Achilles tendons.

9. Up Dog

Lie face down and place your hands on each side of your ribs, tops of the feet down. As you take a breath in and exhale, lift your body up so that your legs lift off the mat as well. You will scoot slightly forward. Draw the shoulder blades back. Look up at the ceiling or straight ahead if you have neck problems. Hold for 10–15 seconds. Rest in child's pose (No.14) to reverse the action of the spine. This pose alleviates stiffness in the shoulders and the lower back, increases energy and is good for posture.

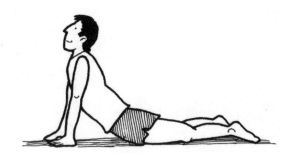

10. Twist

From a seated position, stretch both legs out in front of you. Activate the feet by flexing them and pull one knee up towards your chest. Hug the knee by wrapping the same arm (as the knee that is pulled up) around the knee. Pull straight up in the spine and feel the energy from the bottom of spine up through the crown of the head. As you breathe in, take the free hand and with the palm facing the ear, exhale and raise the hand straight up above your head. Breathe in and out and twist slightly as you allow the hand to come down behind the hip. Hold and breathe. When your body tells you to, walk the hand back into a deeper twist letting it rest behind the opposite hip. Hold for I minute and release. Repeat on the other side. Hug the knee by wrapping the opposite arm around the knee. Count 5–7 breaths and repeat on opposite side.

11. Pigeon

Get into table position (on all fours with your back flat). As you breathe in and exhale, slide one knee forward in between your hands while you allow the other knee to slide out from under you. The front foot moves towards the groin. Lift up high in the spine as you hold for several breaths and then fold over the front knee feeling the lengthening of the spine and outer thighs.

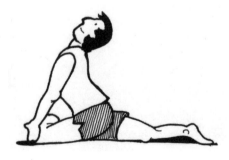

12. Cobbler's Pose

Sit with soles of feet together. If knees are up higher than hip level, sit on cushions high enough to keep knees even with hip level. Rest hands on feet or legs. Keep shoulders relaxed and chest lifted. Count 5–7 breaths. Good hip and groin stretch.

13. Incline

From a seated position and legs straight in front of you, bring your hands along side your hips underneath your shoulders. Rise up on the arms. Try to keep the bottoms of the feet on the ground.

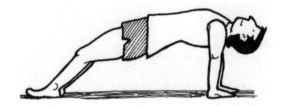

14. Child's Pose

Sit on your heels with your big toes facing each other, knees hip width apart. Fold over the legs as you rest your head on the mat, hands either on each side of the body or stretched out above your head. If this pose puts too much pressure on your head, you can modify either by sitting on a block or by putting a bolster under your head.

15. Boat Pose

Lie on your back. Raise your feet slightly off the mat. Now lift the head and shoulders up as you reach towards your feet with your hands. Short, shallow breaths in through the nose and out through the mouth will help you maintain this posture longer. Long, slow breaths. Also having the knees bent rather than straight will make this pose less difficult. Count 5–7 breaths. This posture strengthens the abdominal, neck and back muscles.

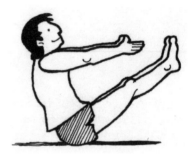

16. Cobra

Lie on your tummy. With elbows bent and close to the body and hands next to your chest, breathe in and exhale as you lift the chest upwards. Be sure to relax the shoulders downward and draw the shoulder blades back. Either look straight ahead or look up to the ceiling. Hold for about 30 seconds and release. Lay on your stomach. Breathe in as you lift the chest upwards. Hold 5–7 breaths. (Depending on the flexibility of your spine you may have to stay down on your forearms, keeping your elbows against your sides.)

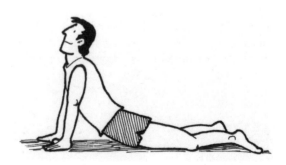

17. Staff

Sit tall with legs extended in front of you with feet flexed. Bring your hands to each side of your hips and push the palm of the hand downward as you lengthen the spine from the base all the way through the crown of your head. Drop the shoulders down and hold. This pose looks easy but is not the easy to hold. Try to hold for 30 seconds.

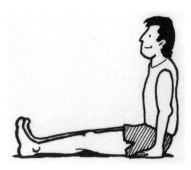

18. Bridge Pose

Lie on your back and bend the knees upward. Lift the hips and begin to walk the shoulders underneath you as you walk your hands under your waist, fingers pointing outward, wrists working towards each other as close as you can get. Relax the throat, breathe and hold for 30 seconds to 1 minute. Release by taking your arms out from under you. Count 5–7 breaths.

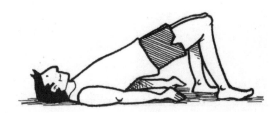

19. Angry Cat

Come onto hands and knees. Hands directly under shoulders and knees hip width apart, tops of the feet on the mat, back in flat position with navel gently pulling in towards spine. Exhale, round the tailbone under, keep navel to spine and round back up towards ceiling. Drop head and slightly tuck in chin. Arms remain straight. Do not shrug shoulders up around back of neck. Continue to breathe. Count 5–7 breaths. Return to flat back position. Do this several times to relieve tightness in back.

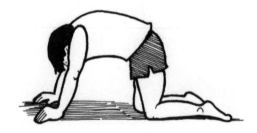

20. Corpse

Gently roll down on your mat on your back. Allow the palms to face up and the feet to release out slightly to the side, legs apart. Tuck the chin in slightly as you feel the neck extend. Now follow your breath and, as you follow your breath, begin to become aware of any tension in your body on your face, in your back, shoulders, legs, hips, etc. Go to these areas and release all tension. As you continue to breathe and release the tension, the mind begins to quieten down as well and you will, over time, be able to go quickly into a deep meditative space within. Practise this pose everyday. You will be glad you did.

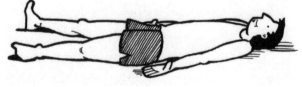

Try to do at least five of these stretches each day, and twice a week, practise all of them. You will be amazed at the results!

AH, LOVELY SLEEP

For some of us happiness comes while we sleep

French Proverb

Sleep is one of the most important needs not just of the body but of the whole self. In our busy lives we are constantly encroaching on our sleeping time. Most of us know we need between seven to nine hours of sleep a night, approximately a third of our lives; however few of us really get enough sleep time and sleep quality. We take it for granted that we can just lie down after a busy day and get good quality, restful sleep and wake up refreshed the next day. There are many reasons why this often doesn't happen and there are also many remedies to help solve the problem.

 It is important to understand that sleep is as valuable a time as anything we do when we are awake. As we strive to achieve and progress we can often view sleep and relaxation as dead time, not just down time. Nothing could be further from the truth.

Just like a business needs to have income to offset its expenditures, we have our own economics called 'the economics of recovery'. This means our need and ability to recover and recuperate. We do this through eating, drinking, relaxing and sleeping but also by being passive and letting go of our concerns and thoughts. To get a good sleep we have to learn to prepare by ending the day properly, switching off our thinking minds, relaxing our bodies and letting go of our worries. It is not always easy but, with practice, it becomes routine and good restful sleep should be the norm. As our life undergoes its upheavals and changes, it is a really good idea to follow these pre-sleep tips to make sure you always get what you need in this department.

1. Maintain a regular bed and waking time schedule including weekends. Our sleep–wake cycle is regulated by a 'circadian clock' in our brain and the body's need to balance both sleep time and wake time. A regular waking time in the morning strengthens the circadian function and can help with sleep onset at night. That is also why it is important

to keep a regular bedtime and waking time, even at weekends when there is the temptation to sleep in.

2. Establish a regular, relaxing bedtime routine such as soaking in a hot tub or bath and then reading a book or listening to soothing music. A relaxing, routine activity right before bedtime conducted away from bright lights helps separate your sleep time from activities that can cause excitement, stress or anxiety which can make it more difficult to fall asleep, get sound and deep sleep or remain asleep. Avoid enlivening activities before bedtime like working, paying bills, engaging in competitive games or family problem solving. Finally, avoid exposure to bright light before bedtime because it signals the neurons that help control the sleep–wake cycle that it is time to wake, not to sleep.

3. Create a sleep-conducive environment that is dark, quiet, comfortable and cool. Design your sleep environment to establish the conditions you need for sleep – cool, quiet, dark, comfortable and free of interruptions. Also make your bedroom reflective of the value you place on sleep. Check your room for noise or other distractions, including a bed partner's sleep disruptions such as snoring, light, and a dry or hot environment. Consider using blackout curtains, eye shades, ear plugs, 'white noise', humidifiers, fans and other devices.

4. Sleep on a comfortable mattress and pillows. Make sure your mattress is supportive. The one you have been using for years may have outlived its life expectancy which is about nine or ten years for most good quality mattresses. Have comfortable pillows and make the room attractive and inviting for sleep but also free of allergens that might affect you and objects that might cause you to slip or fall if you have to get up during the night.

5. Use your bedroom only for sleep and sex to strengthen the association between bed and sleep. It is best to take work materials, computers and televisions out of the sleeping environment If you associate a particular activity or item with anxiety about sleeping, omit it from your bedtime routine. For example, if looking at a bedroom clock makes you anxious about how much time you have before you must get up, move the clock out of sight. Do not engage in activities that cause you anxiety and prevent you from sleeping.

6. Finish eating at least two to three hours before your regular bedtime. Eating or drinking too much may make you less comfortable when settling down for bed. It is best to avoid a heavy meal too close to bedtime. Also, spicy foods may cause heartburn, which can lead to

difficulty falling asleep and discomfort during the night. Try to restrict fluids close to bedtime to prevent visits to the bathroom during the night. However some people find milk or herbal, non-caffeinated teas to be soothing and a helpful part of a bedtime routine.

7. Exercise regularly. It is best to complete your workout at least a few hours before bedtime. In general, exercising regularly makes it easier to fall asleep and contributes to sounder sleep. However, exercising sporadically or right before going to bed will make falling asleep more difficult. In addition to making us more alert, our body temperature rises during exercise, and takes as much as six hours to begin to drop. A cooler body temperature is associated with sleep onset. Finish your exercise at least three hours before bedtime. Late afternoon exercise is the perfect way to help you fall asleep at night.

8. Avoid caffeine (e.g. coffee, tea, soft drinks, colas, chocolate) close to bedtime. It can keep you awake. Caffeine is a stimulant and caffeine products remain in the body on average from three to five hours but they can affect some people for up to twelve hours. Even if you do not think caffeine affects you, it may be disrupting and changing the quality of your sleep. Avoiding caffeine within six to eight hours of going to bed can help improve sleep quality.

9. Avoid nicotine (e.g. cigarettes, tobacco products). Used close to bedtime, it can lead to poor sleep. Nicotine is also a stimulant. Smoking before bed makes it more difficult to fall asleep. When smokers go to sleep, they experience withdrawal symptoms from nicotine, which also causes sleep problems. Nicotine can cause difficulty falling asleep, problems waking in the morning, and may also cause nightmares. Difficulty sleeping is just one more reason to quit smoking. And never smoke in bed or when sleepy!

10. Avoid alcohol close to bedtime. Although many people think of alcohol as a sedative, it actually disrupts sleep, causing nighttime waking. Consuming alcohol leads to a night of less restful sleep.

Source: National Sleep Foundation*

---

*Used with permission of the National Sleep Foundation. For further information, please visit http://www.sleepfoundation.org

THE BENEFITS OF MASSAGE

There isn't nearly enough touch in our world today. Touch is something we crave. It comforts, heals and calms us. Massage is something that satisfies this need but gives us a huge amount of added benefits and, as such, qualifies as a serious necessity for wellbeing. There are almost countless physical as well as emotional benefits to getting regular massage and an abbreviated list follows. It

- Helps relieve stress and aids relaxation

- Helps relieve muscle tension and improves circulation

- Alleviates discomfort during pregnancy

- Fosters faster healing of strained muscles and ligaments

- Reduces pain and swelling and formation of scar tissue

- Provides greater joint flexibility and range of motion

- Enhances athletic performance

- Promotes deeper and easier breathing

- Reduces blood pressure

- Helps relieve tension-related headaches and eye-strain

- Enhances the health and nourishment of skin

- Improves posture

- Strengthens the immune system

- Calms and clears the mind

If you can't afford to hire a therapist or do not have a partner to help out, you can do much of this yourself. Take the time each day to soothe tired muscles with a light self-massage, as well as schedule a regular massage as part of your treating yourself to optimum health and vitality.

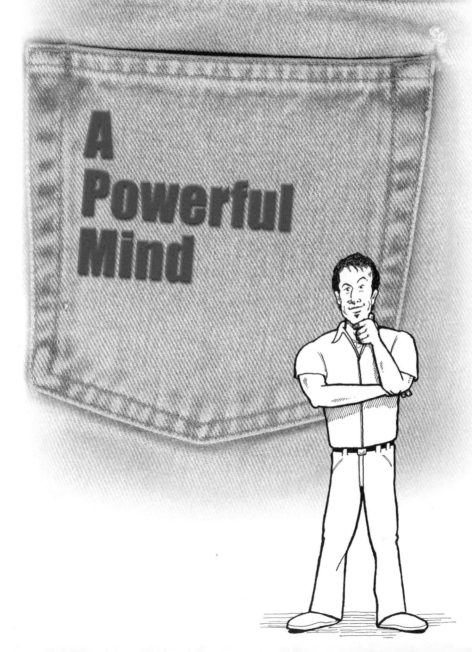

CHAPTER FIVE

A Powerful Mind

MIND POTENTIAL

A dog does not mind being called a dog

African Proverb

Whatever our mind really is, it surely is an amazing tool that allows us to experience the world around us on many levels. We have a lot to think about, react to and make decisions on. Our minds process huge amounts of information, attempt to make sense of it, tag, file and store this information in our memories, make choices and then, hopefully recall the information when needed. Its potential is amazing but it often doesn't work anywhere near its full capability.

This doesn't mean we aren't all doing our best with what we have. It's just that most of us haven't been taught what we are fully capable of and how to train our minds to be sharper and more powerful. One thing for sure is that we all have great potential and are all intelligent in our own way. Our minds are powerful tools and can work as well for us as they can against us. This section is to help you understand your mind better so that you can turn it into more of a friend and workmate rather than something of a limitation and liability. In an ideal world we would have free, versatile, powerful and educated minds. We would be much more likely to be independent and free thinkers, more creative, considerate and dynamic personalities and, I daresay, happier as a result.

Intelligence comes in many forms depending on who we are, how and where we are brought up, what our interests and talents are and what we believe to be true about ourselves and the world we live in. Intelligence is really nothing more than being effective because what good does it do to have knowledge or talent if it cannot be applied and be helpful in some way? Many of us have a great deal of unrealised potential intelligence, skill and talent because we only judge intelligence by cultural standards, past achievements or what our level of general knowledge and skill might be. This is partly due to our own lifestyle choices and lack of ambition but also partly because many of us were told sometime in our past that we are not very bright (book smart), or that we aren't capable of doing this or that. In addition to our past limitations, we may just not have found that thing or subject that interests us enough or really captures our imagination, attention and creative powers to enable us to see what we are capable of. Our minds definitely require interest, motivation and a little confidence to become fully engaged. We have got to give them what they need if we want to use them to their fullest extent.

Attitude

Attitude is everything. You may have heard this before and thought it a little bit of an exaggeration but it is not. Your attitude is the way you see the world, it determines the way you react, your levels of patience and concentration, how much you care, how well you learn and how you stick at things. Ultimately, this all determines how well you do in life and how capable you are of adjusting when things aren't going so well. So, yes, attitude is everything. Not everybody's attitude is good and positive in every situation, every day. We may have a good attitude towards work but a bad one when it comes to exercise or eating right. We may have a good attitude to doing things that will further our goals and career but not so good when someone else asks you to do something. Having a bad attitude is very unhelpful, annoying to all concerned and the single most limiting factor to our potential. We must constantly be prepared to review our attitude to see if it is a help or a hindrance. This book should help you identify your own attitude concerning the main aspects of your life. When you fear or hate some aspect of it, you may be experiencing problems in this area, making it almost impossible to change it for the better. When you love or get excited about another aspect you probably have a good experience and/or are open to ways of making it better because you naturally care more about what you love and enjoy.

The forthcoming sections on positive thinking and affirmations, fear factors and learning from the past, should help you identify the aspects you have a bad attitude about, then show you ways to improve that way of thinking. Just be aware that your life experience depends on your attitude. It is the first thing people see when they meet you and it is the first thing that you use to judge the world around you. A negative attitude makes everything seem negative when it really isn't. We have to do our very best to have a good, open and humble attitude. Don't let a bad attitude hold you back any longer. It is easier than you think to turn it around. A decision to improve this vital aspect of your personality and then a commitment to daily practice is all that is required. Hopefully you will find the methods within these pages.

Learning and Concentration

Knowledge is power. The more we know and apply, the more we are able to shape ourselves, our world and our lives. In order to learn we have to be inspired, motivated and interested. Our minds only concentrate and assimilate information that means something to us, or feel is important to our way of life. The information in this book is very important because it deals with how a person can realise their potential and develop their powers. But to learn this and anything else, we need to be motivated to learn and then apply the information, thus improving ourselves and our situation. A subject must be of significant value to us in the first place or we won't invest the energy or the time to work through it. Our attention and concentration levels are determined largely by our interest and attitude to the subject which, in turn, is affected by our levels of motivation, energy, self-discipline and the general confidence we have in our ability to comprehend it. Concentration is the intensity of the mind's focus on a subject. It requires not only will and desire but also regular practice to develop. Good concentration can be developed by anyone who wants to. Some of the mental and physical exercises laid out in this book can help but, without an interest in learning and a determination to apply ourselves, we never truly realise the learning ability of our minds and their potential to shape our lives.

A HEALTHY MIND

Our minds and bodies are inextricably linked. Simply speaking, this means that they are inseparable and you cannot consider one without the other. Without a healthy body we struggle to think straight, remember clearly, make good and qualified decisions or be patient and effective.

When our minds and emotions are in turmoil our bodies suffer too, displaying symptoms of stress and discomfort that manifest in various physical ways like skin complaints, muscular tension, headaches, weight and hair loss and many other chronic ailments. Equally, we can acquire mental health problems through poor input, i.e. not getting our basic needs met, developing limiting beliefs and by neglecting our bodies. For example, it is very hard to concentrate and think straight when we eat poorly and are regularly dehydrated. Also if we are not happy and comfortable and live in an unsafe or distressing environment we suffer mentally too. Symptoms can range from attention deficit, hyperactivity or personality disorders to depression, anxiety, psychosis and worse. For us to have healthy and well developed minds we first need a healthy body. Once we have begun work on that, we next need to learn more about exactly what a powerful mind requires, what to feed it and how to exercise it. It has amazing capabilities and, just like the body, needs training, maintenance, exercise and rest too. Let's recap on some of the mind's needs so we can get a better idea of this.

Your top ten mind needs

1. **Progress** – We all feel better when we get things done and make progress.

2. **Goals** – They keep our minds focused and productive. Keep them up-to-date and review them regularly.

3. **Organisation** – This is about managing our lives and keeping them in order so that we don't waste time and effort.

4. **Problems/Challenges** – These are necessary irritants to make sure we continue to grow and get stronger.

5. **Achievement** – We all need to accomplish things and feel useful in some way.

6. **Training and Learning** – Your mind is like a muscle. It needs regular and quality training and stimulation to develop and become stronger. Read regularly, problem solve and learn new skills. Languages and music are great for this.

7. **Rules and Boundaries** – Sometimes we need to be disciplined so that we can contain our energies and perform at our best.

8. **Relaxation** – As much as the mind needs to be worked it needs to relax and stop thinking. Take time to be quiet or read something that takes you away from your daily reality. Learn to be more passive and let things come to you. Stretching routines and meditation are great for mental relaxation.

9. **Non-attachment** – We are not our possessions or our thoughts. We must constantly learn to let go.

10. **Humour** – See the funny side regularly and don't take life too seriously all the time.

In addition to these needs we also have other requirements to stimulate and develop our minds fully, including:

- **Social Interaction** – We all need social contact and feedback from others.

- **Communication** – Speak your mind but try to get better at communicating clearly, compassionately and purposefully.

- **Debate** – Learn to be able to stick up for yourself verbally and make your point calmly and firmly.

- **Facts/Data** – Be informed so you know what you are dealing with.

- **Novelty** – A regular injection of new is good for you, but don't just change for the sake of it.

- **Recognition** – We all need to be recognised for our achievements and individuality. Make sure you respect that in others too.

- **Mystery** – It would be boring if we knew everything. Stay curious and explore often.

- **Responsibility** – Identify and take care of your responsibilities. You are only responsible for your own life. You can help others but take care of your own business first.

- **Optimism** – Practice staying positive.

- **Practice** – Makes perfect. Enjoy any practice you do. It really does work and is worth the effort.

- **Prospects** – We all need to create prospects for ourselves as well as being open to ones that come along. It is important to have things to look forward to.

- **Loss** – You only own your body and your time, be prepared to let everything else go.

- **Reflection** – Take time to reflect and appreciate what happened in the past. Always use a positive attitude towards the past.

- **Grounding** – Prioritising, staying in touch with nature and what really matters keeps us all grounded and balanced.

- **Pleasure** – Remember life is to be enjoyed as much as possible. Pleasure is always heightened after work and achievement.

- **Instruction** – Learn to take a little instruction, you may not know everything after all.

- **Rules** – It is important to know the rules beforehand. Set some for yourself to keep yourself in check.

- **Closure** – You have to be able to properly finish something before you can begin something else.

- **Reward** – We all need reward for our efforts. This can come in many forms and should be good and not harmful to us.

- **Discipline** – Hones and polishes us.

- **Observation** – Be more aware of what is going on around you and stay observant. We all miss far too much.

- **Routine/Consistency** – Life is and should be very rhythmic. Routine and consistency is the vital backbone of progress.

- **Spontaneity** – Don't be afraid to shake things up from time to time.

- **Questioning** – If something doesn't sit right with you, then question it. Don't believe everything you are told and read.

- **Interests** – A varied life is a fulfilling one.

- **Feedback** – Listen to what others have to say.

Think about which needs you miss out on and the activities you could do more or less of to get them back in your life.

OWNING YOUR MIND

When you have a well-developed and powerful mind, you are a more powerful person with a greater awareness of what is going on, plus a better memory and keener intuition and instincts (hindsight and foresight), resulting in more confidence in your abilities. As we develop our powers we must also make sure that we maintain ownership of our minds and not let ourselves get too influenced and conditioned by others' agendas and ideals. When we have a good knowledge of what makes us tick and know ourselves sufficiently to know what is good for us, we are much more likely to make choices that are more beneficial to our health and overall happiness. If our minds are underdeveloped and weak and we have less self-awareness and knowledge of how the world works, then we are much more easily undersold, influenced and even brainwashed to our inevitable detriment. We do need to be open to different views, but sometimes we have to protect ourselves from those who want to sell us products and ideas that are not good for us. Unfortunately not everyone has our best interests at heart. The stronger our mind and identity becomes the better we become at rooting out this kind of stuff. It is not always easy to decipher the truth behind everything we see, but this is where our deeper senses like our conscience, authenticity, imagination and intuition come in. We all have these powerful tools at our disposal and they help us to know what is right for us and those around us. A strong and independent mind is more able to project consequences and possible future outcomes. We can avoid a lot of trouble this way. By being powerful and independent we maintain a good grip on our own minds and protect our freedoms.

Know yourself, listen to your conscience, use your imagination and be true to yourself.

THE CREATIVE PROCESS

A major aspect of our mental power is our ability to create. We discussed in the beginning of the book the notion that we have the ability to create much of our own reality and manifest our ideas. Let's expand on that and see how it all works. We seldom realise that our ideas and desires have an energy of their own. Our ideas are just pure energy waiting to be developed into real things and events through our creative powers. All humans have this capability of taking a thought or idea and making it become something real. Just think of all the fabulous inventions that people have come up with through the ages; most of them were normal people just like you and me who had an interest in something, a good idea and the desire to see it become reality. With so many different ideas to improve so many different things using so many different methods, one thing always remained a constant; as humans we all create in roughly the same way. We seem to follow a set recipe or process. This process is part of the fabric of nature itself and we use it instinctively any time we want to make or create anything. It is the natural way an idea becomes reality and teaches us a great deal about how our mind can operate on different levels.

We all know that we cannot get something from nothing and create things out of fresh air. Well, maybe David Copperfield or Ali Bongo can, but the majority of us have to follow certain rules, work hard and smart and follow instructions and blueprints if we are to achieve a desired result. What I am saying here is that, if there is a need and you have a good idea to satisfy that need, good intentions and are prepared to work hard, then you have much of what is required to manifest what you want. So did all the great inventors of history but they also knew they had to follow the universal creative process. It is the process that turns an idea into actual living and working reality. It is the necessary stepped process we all have to follow if we want to bring an idea to life. Some would call it magic. I just think it's natural when you know how it works.

Let's start with the basics. Everything is energy at its fundamental level. For an idea, which initially is pure energy and only exists in your mind as a thought pattern, to become something real and solid, there must be a gradual process similar to deciding to bake a cake and then going about baking it. You have nothing in the beginning but a desire but then, through a process, you make something. It takes steps and these steps always follow a specific pattern as the desire becomes an idea, a plan, a collection of ingredients and tools, a mixture, and so on until it is put in the oven, baked, eaten and enjoyed. The interesting thing is that it takes the same number and type of steps each time, beginning with the need and ending with the result. I need a cake, I make it and I eat it, resulting in a full tummy and a smile on my face. This is the universal creative process and it is how the mind manifests things. With this creative process explained, hopefully you will understand a little more about your mind's capabilities, how it works on different levels and how we can adjust these modes of thought at will, depending on what type of thinking is best for any given situation. But first let's look at how all these clever inventors and creative people used the process and outline exactly how it works so you can learn how to make it work for you. First everything begins not with an idea exactly, but with a need (ever heard the phrase 'necessity is the mother of invention'?). So this is where we get the initial idea as a reaction to the need we feel. Once we have our idea, we use our imagination to make a judgment as to whether it is a good idea and whether or not to take action. We balance up the pros and cons of the situation. If we decide to act on our idea the next phase is to create an ideal plan or design to make it a reality. Once we have a plan, recipe or design, the next phase is to figure out all the ingredients and tools that we are going to need. The next step is to put it all together, to organise these ingredients and begin to form something out of them. This is the real making or construction phase. It is the performance part of the creative process. Next, we test it to see if it works or decide on any changes that are needed. Once all this is done, finally we have our idea in its manifest, physical form. If we had a good idea and design, quality ingredients, organised everything properly, made it and tested it well, then it will probably be a good and useful product. The lesson here is that we can turn our ideas into reality and we do this every day without realising this ideal process exists. But if we want an ideal result then we need to follow this recipe and respect the creative process. In this physical world there are certain rules to follow and these are the ones of creative manifestation. Any aspects missed and the result is different and inferior. Just like the baking of a cake, we all have to follow a recipe if we want a great result. This shows us how, ultimately, we have a kind of 'mind over matter' influence on our lives and our environment. That is why we have so much potential power and we must be careful with this power and use it wisely. It doesn't have to be an important invention. It might just be your own and your family's life that you are influencing with your creative powers. Be conscious of your capability to affect the world around you. Use your powers wisely!

Recap:

1. Idea

2. Judgment/Choice

3. Design/Plan

4. Ingredients/Tools

5. Form/Organise/Practise

6. Performance

7. Result/Effect

This is the creative process, the difference between just wishing and actually making something happen. For good and for bad we follow the same basic recipe. We need to use our imagination when deciding whether an idea is a good one or not. It never has to go beyond the judgment stage if we can see that the consequence isn't going to be helpful and constructive. One of the most amazing things about our minds is their capability to follow an idea to its potential conclusion just through the use of imagination. This is what we call our judgment and the healthier and better informed we are, the better and more successful judgments we tend to make. So learn to use this tool more effectively. You can save a great deal of time and resources by planning it all in your mind and on paper first. If it passes this test then it may be worth moving on to the design phase and organisational phase. Just make sure it is worth it and follow the ideal creative process.

POSITIVE THINKING

One of the reasons why we become negative sometimes and lose our motivation and enthusiasm is because we let life drag us down and get into the habit of thinking negatively and limiting ourselves. When we allow ourselves to develop a negative attitude it is the most common recurring obstacle to us really being who we can be and doing the things we want to do. Our attitude is the projection of the thoughts, beliefs and expectations we have from our life and the world in general. To change our attitude we have to change the way we think and adjust some of our negative beliefs and expectations. We are like magnets in this world; the more positive we are, the more positive our experience seems to be. Many of us are attracting our difficulties and painful experiences and we don't even know it. It is possible to make these changes. It just takes a little practice, and of course, a little positive thinking.

We all know how our negativity can badly affect us and we have all experienced how a positive attitude can see us through difficult times plus make the most of opportunities when they come along. This section is about how to get into a more positive frame of mind more of the time and not let our weaker side drag us down so much. We dig a lot of the holes we find ourselves in and we have to learn how to stop the self sabotage. Instead of being dynamic and believing in ourselves and using negative experiences as lessons to become stronger, we allow negative feelings and beliefs to develop and often these become ingrained as part of our thinking, mostly because we spend so much time dwelling on them. We need to understand that our life experiences, the way our body feels and performs, situations that happen in our career, relationships, etc. are greatly determined by our attitude, our beliefs, by how we think and react. All of these can be changed for the better.

You've probably heard the phrase 'seeing is believing'. Actually, the opposite is true. If first you believe, then you will see. Negative thoughts and beliefs will only bring negative reactions and situations and sap your energy. You don't need to be at the mercy of these destructive beliefs and attitudes. You can detach yourself from them and instead choose to relate to a positive and more hopeful view and react in a more positive way. It is not easy but with practice it is like achieving any new skill; practice makes perfect. Everything that happens to us is an opportunity for learning and growth. If we can learn to react in a more positive way then we are more likely to see a positive outcome from the situation. This is our attitude at work and it spreads, depending on how we use it. For example, if you hear yourself saying, "I always feel so stressed on a Monday morning" or "I always get so nervous in front of a group of people" or "It's so hard for me to lose weight" or "I always gain the weight back that I've lost", you are expressing your limiting beliefs. Your beliefs dictate your experience! When you repeat negative thoughts habitually, they become your beliefs and you project these negative and often inaccurate beliefs on to other aspects of your life. The amazing thing is that this really is just a choice on your part. You know you can think and react differently, in a more positive way and be a magnet for better things. This is a choice you have to make before any previous negativity can be undone.

When you decide to make a change in your attitude, you must first analyse the beliefs you are carrying around about yourself and the world around you. As an exercise, try writing down the things you believe to be true about yourself but would like to change. Become aware of what you say to yourself and to others about the way you are. For example, you might say, "I wish I could improve my endurance levels, but I've never had good energy levels and I get tired easily". Watch out for those words 'always' and 'never', especially when they are used in a negative context. Beliefs like this make it almost impossible to change things for the better. Try this. As soon as you hear something negative, think of a more positive response, such as:

- **Negative response** – I know I'll never play my best game vs.
  Positive response – I know if I keep practising and believe in myself, the performances will come.

- **Negative response** – I can never relax vs.
  Positive response – I know if I keep working hard at my yoga and relaxation exercises, I will become more relaxed and sleep better.

Even if you feel as though you're not telling the truth, the interesting thing about a lie is that if you repeat it enough you begin to believe it. If you dwell on your past, your focus on the present will suffer and your goals may slip farther away. This, to a large extent, is how you reinvent yourself. Along with carrying out the required tasks and taking care of the 'to do's', you have to support these with the appropriate kind of thinking and attitude. When you combine positive thought with positive action you become an almost irresistible magnet for success and wellbeing. Make an effort every day to reprogramme your thoughts into positive messages. If you are consistent in your efforts, you will be rewarded with a more joyful, balanced and satisfying life.

INSPIRATIONS AND AFFIRMATIONS

Can't think of anything positive to say about yourself? Don't know where to look to find a quotation or inspirational message that speaks to you? All you need to do is to go to these sections in your Life Coach and make a selection for your day. A couple of things should be remembered. Your mind is waiting for you to adopt a positive or negative tone for the day. This is why it is so important to start it with a hopeful and positive mantra (mental exercise). Some that seem the most difficult to apply to our lives may be the ones most needed and so, repeating them diligently, will only serve to bring us closer to knowing ourselves more deeply. How many times have we read things that made us think, "That is so true. That's exactly what I believe" or "Oh, yes, I've read that book. Wasn't it great? It really makes you think!" Well, that's all just wonderful, but the problem is, even though you say you agree with it or believe the things it says and it does make you think, you don't put it into practice in your daily life. It might make you think but what do you ever do about it? Use it or lose it? Absolutely! These wonderful books of endless information are not just fairy tales to tickle the imagination. These quotes and inspirational messages are not just great car stickers and greeting cards. They are actually tools and if you follow what they say, you will experience some wonderful results. The best thing is that, the more you practice, the better life gets. Begin your day with positive thoughts and end it with appreciation and thanks.

Examples:

- I trust myself to know what is good for me.

- I understand that I must take care of myself first before I can effectively take care of anyone or anything else.

- I realise there are no mistakes in my life, rather, only lessons I must learn.

- I will accomplish a simple act or thought of kindness towards someone in my life.

- I promise myself I will ask for guidance when I feel I need it.

- I take time each day to be outdoors with nature.

- I know that when I release anger, fear, sadness and frustration I allow space for positive things to come into my life.

- I take steps to find activities that will be fun and improve my wellbeing.

- I read a book or listen to an audiotape that teaches and inspires me to take care of myself at least once a month.

- I will say only positive things when I look into the mirror

- I am a very accomplished golfer/gardener/teacher/student.

Think like you want to be.

YOUR PERSONAL AFFIRMATIONS

This is one of the most important mental aspects of life coaching. Until you get used to thinking like a person who expects to realise their goals and dreams, you must make an act of it. In this case, practise the thinking with an affirmation exercise. You have learned how to be more positive now, so get into the practice of saying it. Just as getting fit requires training and routine practice, so does positive thinking and affirmations. Now that you are changing your daily routine and creating new habits with improved actions you must keep your mind up to speed. Any time during the day you can repeat these messages to yourself but it's especially important in the morning or when you feel stressed, anxious or depressed. Look at some of the examples from Positive Thinking and weigh those up against your goals and how you feel you would like to progress, and say it as if it was your reality today. It is good to begin with your name and a basic mission statement like, "I want love, peace, wisdom and success in my life". Then move on to the key affirmations that you feel will help to forge the strong and positive new beliefs and expectations that you are wishing for. Mean what you say and respect this practise as though it is a ritual. It is always nice to close the day with something like, "I appreciate everything that has happened today, I appreciate all I have, the people, my material comforts. I acknowledge that I did the best I could today and leave all my worries to a higher power. I let the day go and with it any mistakes or regret, sadness and guilt that I may have felt". Here is a space for you to write in and practice your daytime affirmations. Change it when you feel the need.

- My name is ...   and I want love, peace, wisdom and success in my life. I am healthy, strong and positive. I am free from fear and negativity.
- I find it easy to ...   e.g. get going on a Monday.
- I feel fit and relaxed and very positive about my prospects.
- I enjoy ...
  e.g. working hard toward my goals.
- I feel stronger every day
- Nothing gets me down for long
- I appreciate my family and friends
- I appreciate my health and lovely home
- I am lucky to have ...
- I will sleep well and wake up refreshed tomorrow morning ready for another great day ahead

You decide the exact words. Try writing them on a piece of card and keep it beside your bed to read when you wake up and before you go to sleep. Make your affirmations the first thing you do and your appreciations the last. Practise this and soon it will become habit and normal thinking. Use the following pages to create your own affirmation exercise. It really works!

Create your own weekly affirmations and get into the practice of thinking positively.

Monday ....

....

....

Tuesday ....

....

....

Wednesday ....

....

....

Thursday ....

....

....

Friday ....

....

....

Saturday ....

....

....

Sunday ....

....

....

Comments: ....

....

....

Monday ....

....

....

Tuesday ....

....

....

Wednesday ....

....

....

Thursday ....

....

....

Friday ....

....

....

Saturday ....

....

....

Sunday ....

....

....

Comments: ....

....

....

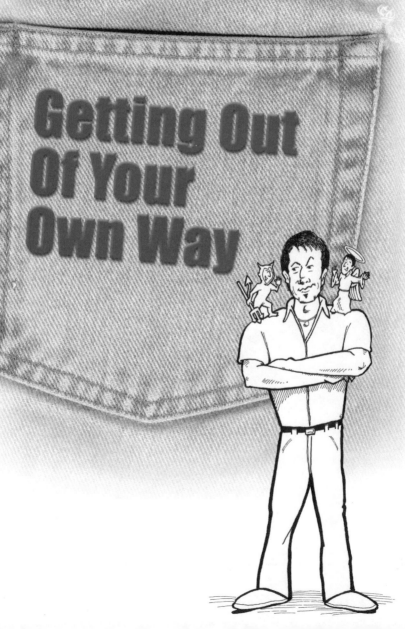

CHAPTER SIX

Getting Out Of Your Own Way

YOUR OWN WORST ENEMY

How many corners do I have to turn, how many times do I have to learn, all the love I have is in my mind?

The Verve

You really are your own worst enemy; we all are. We judge ourselves so harshly and so often talk to ourselves in a mean and condescending way. We are very slow to remember our past successes and to forgive our past mistakes, yet we are extremely quick to criticise our efforts and allow ourselves to feel inferior to others. What we are really talking about here is how much we love ourselves and, subsequently, how easy or hard we are on ourselves as a result. The harder we are, the more difficult it is to have real joy in our lives, for the simple reason that we are not allowing ourselves to feel joy, success and progress. You may already have an idea as to how this became part of your thinking and there is more to cover in the later section on learning from the past. The question here is simple and one you must address if your real potential is going to be allowed to blossom: are you going to forgive yourself all your shortcomings, learn from the past, accept yourself, and move forward with an attitude of love and respect for yourself or are you going to continue to be your own worst enemy? The answer and the resulting freedom and confidence that will inevitably arise from it is a decision that only you can make. We all look for validation and love from others but it is from within ourselves that we have to find the love, forgiveness and permission to be happy, healthy and successful. We all deserve this, but we often don't all allow it to become a reality.

 We all need to forgive, release, accept, love, appreciate and GET ON WITH ENJOYING OUR LIVES!

FEAR FACTORS

Fear gets in the way a lot. Fear is natural when it is rational, when there is a good reason to be afraid. Some fears are very helpful too. You may have a fear of gambling or drugs because you don't want to introduce them into your life through a fear they might become destructive. You may be afraid of driving too fast because you may have been in an accident because you or someone else was driving recklessly. Now you drive very steadily and safely because of that fear. These are basically helpful fears. Then there are the irrational, unfounded fears and many of our problems are caused by these.

We create a lot of our own problems by allowing ourselves to become unbalanced, lose our perspective and healthy attitude and by putting unnecessary pressure on ourselves. We seldom realise that we don't have to let this happen. When we attach ourselves to our fears, just as we can with other negative emotions such as guilt, anger and regret, we become them and they become us. They limit and often paralyse our ability to choose, act and make changes for the better. The anxiety and fear levels in the world today are rising not falling. Granted this has a lot to do with crazy people in positions of power and the by-products of a purely gain and profit oriented economy but, ultimately, it is up to us as individuals to decide how much fear we CHOOSE to acknowledge, accept and react to. When we are healthy, balanced and confident, which we all have the power to be, fear becomes less of a factor and we become freer, braver and more purpose and wellbeing driven. With fear we withdraw, become discouraged and conserve. With the opposite mindset of enthusiasm, love, acceptance and hope we expand, encourage and explore.

Most of our fears are an illusion, a perceived pressure that we allow to oppress us. We are freer than we think and potentially immune to the irrational fear that continues to consume us one by one, family by family and community by community. It is our own psychology, attitudes and beliefs that dictate our relative levels of happiness and calm, fear or distress. We get so used to thinking negatively and choosing fear instead of love and appreciation that, even though we have all we need to be healthy and happy, we choose to dwell on our inadequacies, what others have that we don't or what problems and disasters might occur tomorrow. So much of life these days causes us fear and anxiety. We are bombarded each day with reasons to be afraid. We don't have enough money, we might get fired, the new terrorist threat is upon us or there is a new disease about to break out that might kill us all. It is easy to get caught up in all of this and carry a high level of anxiety around with us as a result. Some of it is real but so much of it is not. We must try actively to resist becoming victims of this scaremongering. Let go of as much fear as possible and focus on being as positive, loving and relaxed as possible. Alternatively, maybe it is time we asked ourselves; "Are all my fears real?" and "Can I let go of some of my fears?" The answer to this is a hearty YES! Our happiness as well as our levels of fear and anxiety are all states of mind that we have been conditioned to think and feel over time. We can change these attitudes and thought habits as you have already learned when it comes to positive thinking.

At various times in our lives it becomes pertinent to re-examine the contents of our minds and hearts to determine if they are good and helpful or not. Maybe it is time for a clear out? Through a determined change of attitude, time, practice and patience with yourself, you can significantly lessen the negative impact that fear has on your health and life in general. You have to decide which fears are truly merited and are actually helpful and which are downright harmful to you and holding you back because you habitually dwell on them. If you are afraid of dying young from cancer or another disease and a lifestyle change will help you release some of this fear, then this is a positive action you can take. You may have a fear of debt, so let go of some of your materialistic ways and cut your expenses. You may have a fear of death and this may be holding you back from really living each day to the full. All of these fears need assessing and bringing into the light of day either to be acted on or let go. It might be comforting to know that so many of your fears that are causing you real discomfort and pose future health hazards are those that you can release but it is often easier to keep them rather than facing them because they are so familiar and habitual. As with anything else worthwhile, it requires a little effort, patience, practice, courage and perseverance and we can all become free of irrational and limiting fear.

Saying Good-bye to Constant Fear and Anxiety

Obstacles are those frightful things we see when we lose sight of our goals

Henry Ford

Some fears are not that limiting, scary or so tough to let go of. If you have a fear of heights then not going up in tall buildings or climbing trees won't ruin your life. But fear of speaking to a group when your job requires it, or fear of talking to your loved one about an emotional or personal issue, or fear of failure in a certain thing that stops you enjoying it or even fear of success which often brings on premature and unnecessary failure, do need to be addressed, understood, made light of and let go. Take your time with this section. Don't be afraid to let fear know it isn't going to rule certain aspects of your life any more. Some days you are more confident and courageous than others. Try to work through this section when you are feeling particularly strong and positive, you will see things much more clearly and objectively. Your fear will be there for you to identify but it will be easier for you to rationalise and understand. Each time you make sense of a fear you diminish its power over you. Identify it, ask yourself where it came from and accept that you feel that way but detach from it and let it go. Remember, it is your decision to maintain an attachment to this. (It may be helpful to get a little feedback from a trusted and rational friend or family member on this one.) With practice you will become free of this fear and further unlock your potential.

Write down your fears, whatever they might be. Ask yourself in what way they limit you and then decide whether you can let them go or not. Ask yourself this; If you are fed up with fears, anxiety and worries ruining your life, how much of your time do you spend in fear and on worry, and how much time do you think you have left in this life? You may find that you are choosing to dwell on negatives more than you are actually living and doing positive things. None of us lives forever and none of us is guaranteed to be here even the day after tomorrow. So focus on how you want to think and live – live every moment as a celebration of your life and stop allowing your fears to dominate your world. Lay as many of them aside as you can and hopefully some of them for good!

Let go of as much as you can. Most of them are either not important or redundant anyway.

Fear	Limitation	Solution

THE DARK SIDE

We all have a bit of a dark side or 'shadow personality'. We try to be sweetness and light most of the time but sometimes we are moody, selfish, impatient, greedy, hurtful and deceitful. Our dark side can be downright scary and quite destructive at times too. Just when you think your darker nature is nothing but an out of control, wrecking ball with nothing positive to come from it, you find that, if you look hard enough, something positive and creative always comes from a brush with your dark side. You can learn to be lighter and say farewell to your more destructive and dangerous aspects.

For so much of our history we have been fighting the 'forces of darkness' as our feared enemy. Sometimes it is an outside force that we have deemed threatening to our personal, communal or national safety, but more often it is the demons within us that we have the most desperate battles with. Just as with any other perceived danger or obstacle, it is only our lack of understanding that causes us to react poorly to the problem together with the amount of time we spend worrying about it. Trying to control or eliminate it only gives it more power and significance. When you understand your dark side better it becomes so much easier to deal with. Under pressure you may have a tendency to be aggressive and want to fight people and the world in general. You might be the type who berates yourself harshly for mistakes or disappointments which you think are all your fault. Whether you become over critical with yourself or others, angry, guilty, mean and spiteful inwardly or outwardly, this dark nature is only prevalent because you have lost your balance, joy, love and acceptance. We all have to deal with annoying situations and we are all a little down on ourselves at times, but the battles that we wage within and without are often so unnecessary. Sometimes it becomes the norm to be fighting constantly. It may be a novel concept to you but as long as we maintain our balance, strength and personal harmony, the battles become fewer and farther between, the enemies look more like friends and the storms become more of a gentle breeze. So it ultimately comes down to a choice for us again.

We are free to spend as much time as we want battling with our enemies and dwelling on our own shortcomings and weaknesses or we can decide to focus on being as empowered, enlightened and positive as possible. By bringing more light into our lives, we banish the dark, not through aggression and struggle but through understanding, love and positive action. The fight between good and evil is the oldest drama we have, even older than *Coronation Street* or *General Hospital*. Mostly it goes on in our own minds. When we are unhealthy and unhappy we struggle with ourselves and inevitably this spills out into mean and destructive behaviour. We will always be given the choice between doing something that is good for us and those around and that which is destructive. As long as we are strong and happy in ourselves this choice isn't too difficult to make. We will always choose the positive course if we are in our right minds and this is the abiding lesson. Maintain your own light (wisdom) and warmth (love) and you will usually be loving and productive as an individual. Allow regret, confusion, fear and self-loathing to creep into your system and the demon wrecking ball will have its chaotic way. We have no control over outside forces, we can only do the best with what we have. We still have the choice. As old as this lesson is, we still have the free will and the resources to prevail. The question is, "Will your light and love shine through?"

BLACK AND WHITE THINKING

Life comes at us in full colour; it is more than just black and white. When we become narrow minded we tend to think either in one way or the opposite. We have talked about expanding our awareness and being less narrow minded but it is important to see what kind of limited thinking we can get into. Let us call this black and white thinking. It is very limiting in that it lacks perspective and leaves us few options and a rigid attitude. We need to be flexible in this colourful and contrasting world both physically and mentally so black and white, either/or thinking just doesn't work very well. For example, we might have an opinion which we believe to be right yet someone else has an opposing view which they believe in just as strongly. Rather than thinking that one must be right and the other wrong, we must accept the possible validity of the opposing viewpoint even though it is contrary to our own.

Black and white thinking is either right (if we like it) or wrong (if we don't like or understand it). We categorise people and things as good or bad, right or wrong, depending on our immediate reaction, without considering that there might be another perspective. We might say that all of a certain type, or race, or sex, or age group or religion is always this or that way. We might make other huge generalisations that not only limit our possibility for positive relationships, but genuinely put others off having one with us. We can also develop black and white thinking in relation to ourselves. We say things like, "Well if I can't complete that diet or project then I there's no point in ever trying that again." Just because you couldn't make it work one way doesn't mean you can't make it work another. Often this internal battle comes about because we struggle to stay reasonable and balanced in our thinking, especially toward ourselves when so much emotion is involved. I know it is easier said than done, but if you can try to take as much emotion out of the subject as possible and not go to too much of an extreme, you may have a chance to imagine other possibilities and solutions. If one method is deemed useless, try not to react with the exact opposite view. We must find harmony between our two basic natures, our animal/emotional and our intellectual/mental if we are to break the pattern of black and white thinking.

We are intelligent and sensitive people in need of achievement, giving, purpose, love and compassion but remember that we are still animals. We must have certain physical needs and desires met, so we can be very self-centred at times. The way forward for us is to live a more considered and compassionate life inwardly and outwardly, one that is more sustainable and geared toward satisfying our true nature, our true needs. We can accomplish this in our modern world. We just have to be dynamic and accepting, with a healthy 'give and take' attitude, think laterally and appreciate another's point of view. This is our true nature, we are programmed to be givers as well as takers. We cannot change the world on our own individually, we can only change the way we are as individuals. So find your balance and be considerate in everything you do and don't be so reactive and polarised in the way you think. We have a full spectrum of views that allow us to consider all aspects of an experience and we must employ these powers more consciously if we want to be more effective and realise our potential.

We do indeed have opposite sides to our character but this is no black and white, either/or divide despite how it may seem. They are two sides of the same coin, a spectrum of character that, at the opposing poles, seem at odds but are very much connected as they blend and connect to form our whole personality. Within our full capacity we find individual perspectives that enable us to view the world on all levels relevant to our lives, in full colour as it were. This is where our thinking mind joins with our senses in perceiving and making sense of everything on as many levels as we can. When we are healthy, strong and clear minded, we are better at using our different perspectives to our advantage.

DIFFERENT PERSPECTIVES AND THE DYNAMIC MIND

Sometimes we seem to have only one viewpoint but we do have many mental tools to choose from and all of us have used this range of perspectives at some time or other. Our problems come when we get stuck in one particular perspective and ignore others that might be better and more helpful. For example, if we are very physically oriented we might get fixated on a part of our bodies without appreciating the health of the whole. If, in general we are body obsessed without enough intellectual or spiritual stimulation for our other side, we can develop an imbalance that causes disorders and addictions which can become hazardous to our health. We may be obsessed with how much money we make and work too hard at the expense of our family and friends. On the other hand, we can sometimes go the other way and become too non-materialistic and forget to pay enough attention to our bills and physical wellbeing. Some people spend too much time on intellectual endeavours and forget to exercise or sleep enough. Sometimes we can overreact to an unbalanced lifestyle and, through our attempts to get healthier, renounce our physical and personal comforts and habits in favour of a strict and ascetic spiritual lifestyle. This may bring problems of its own. Remember, health and wellbeing is all about balance and harmony. An unbalanced mind affects us in so many ways. Our relationships often struggle when we don't appreciate another's mindset at a particular time and become too stubborn to change our own for the sake of harmony. For example we might get frustrated and upset with our partner if they put a dampener on our dreams because they are thinking more practically. You may have been thinking about having fun after work but they have spent all day worrying about problems at their job and are in no mood for what you have in mind. This illustrates how differing perspectives can make communication difficult. It takes a dynamic, open and balanced mind to be able to change your view so that you can see things in a constructive, considered and reasonable way. The real lesson here is that we have these different perspectives available to us but we have to get more used to using them when we need to. This is the key to being a more empathetic and ultimately more reasonable person and to more harmonious and effective living.

The freer we are of physical tension, which decreases the mind's ability to be flexible (see stretching section), the more balanced our life is and the more likely we are to be dynamic and make better choices. We can have it both ways. We can be clear and principled for ourselves but we can be equally dynamic and considerate of another's perspective and views. We can be deeply spiritual and highly intellectual people and, at the same time, enjoy our bodies and physical pleasures, as well as being a little naughty and childlike at times. We can take a lot and give a lot too.

Life isn't a test to see who can give or accumulate the most and it is a fact that nobody in this world is perfect. Life is about finding your own personal happiness, wellbeing and direction and then sharing what you have with others. We can have our material comforts as well as being active in charities. We can be creative and have a great sense of humour as well as being tough and capable of undergoing hardship. The lesson here is not to allow yourself to get lopsided and narrow minded by living a narrow existence. By developing a fulfilling, healthy and balanced lifestyle you will get used to using your full array of 'thinking heads' (perspectives) and senses. Then, naturally, you will have the mental, physical and emotional tools to make the best of your life and positively affect those around you.

LEARNING FROM THE PAST

Like it or not, come what may, the past makes us what we are today. The past forms part of our programming and greatly influences our decision making today, which, in turn determines what new history we will make for ourselves tomorrow. Many, if not all, of us have had traumatic and painful things happen to us in our past and will no doubt have more to come. Loss, disappointment and pain are a part of life. We all experience things that have rocked us and shaped and seasoned us but we are still here. The main thing is it hasn't killed us. We deal with it and we move on, but some of us have a harder time moving on than others. We all have bad and painful memories and we often have the physical scars to show for them too. It is how we let this affect us now and in the future that is the main focus of this section. Memories are very useful to us but they can be limiting and destructive too. Our 'world view' and attitude is greatly affected by what has happened to us in the past. If we have seen and felt a lot of pain, lies and cruelty, then we are more likely to believe the world is a cruel and painful place to live. Conversely if we have experienced mostly honesty, integrity, love and encouragement, we are likely going to see the world in quite a different light.

What we choose to remember from our past goes a long way to determining our attitude and reaction to our world. This may have to change if it has become negative and limiting for you. We all have our familiar emotions that we seem to associate with as a result of some of our past experiences. Some people are very joyous and positive by nature and some are skeptical and pessimistic. Whatever nature you are, if it works for you and you find life relatively satisfying and hopeful, you get along with most people and cope with inevitable disappointment and loss when they arise, then you are well adjusted and are more likely to make the most of your life. If however you are easily angered, are often frustrated or constantly seem to carry around a feeling of guilt or sadness then you might be in need of reconciling some of your past and adjust your thinking about it to help support the positive progress you are making on other fronts. The idea here is to learn what you can from the past, put it into a healthy perspective and then let go of what pain and negativity you can while remembering the successes and good times more. As a result of some aspects of your past you might find yourself saying, "I am angry", or "I am so guilty about this or that", or "She made me feel this frustrated" and with plenty of time of dwelling on the matter you become gradually more immersed in that painful emotion. You become it and it becomes you. It is amazing how much you are holding on to and you don't realise that you are deciding to do it consciously.

You must understand that the past pain you hold on to is actually somewhat of a choice. As painful and real as it still feels, you are largely in control of how much of that pain and negativity stays with you or you let go. You may never fully forget the things that happened to you and that is OK. Memories are tools, they help us and shape us but we often choose to dwell on them more than is good for us sometimes. You have to get out of the habit of dredging up and immersing yourself in painful memories and their associated emotions and practise forgiveness and letting go of them instead. Just as you are learning other exercises in this book to help you strengthen yourself and release tension and pain, this is an exercise that you must practice if you are to succeed in breaking free of the ties that have bound and limited you to this point. To begin, start by writing down names of emotions like anger, sadness, regret, frustration, etc., and see what comes to mind. Think of people who you feel have hurt you and write them down. Think of situations that were painful and write them down. You may end up with quite a collection and it may be emotional but when you have them in front of you ask yourself if you want to keep the painful emotions as part of your life, would you like to maintain the fear and anger etc., or would you like to let it go? The same goes for any time you feel that someone or something limited you and you believed in the limits placed on you. Free yourself from these limitations, they are most likely not true; you just allowed yourself to believe them and became associated with those negative and limiting thoughts. Is this your genuine reality or are these just a collection of unfortunate and unfair situations that you, for whatever reason, couldn't shake and simply got used to?

It really is your choice, once you have reconciled these painful, past events, to still carry them around with you. It's as simple as that. You know more now about how limiting beliefs work to hold you back. If you think it is too hard and beyond your control, then it is; that is your reality that you have created by your beliefs and expectations. But if you take the attitude that if you give yourself permission to let it/them go and remind yourself that it comes down to a simple choice and regular practice, then you are half way there. This book really is about reinventing yourself and if you are indeed serious about that, if you really do want a better life for yourself and develop your strengths while letting go of your weaknesses and baggage, then this is as important as any other positive action. Lighten the load and shed your skin. Breathe in the fresh air of freedom.

Recap:

- You are not your emotions, learn to control them.

- You can let go of past pain and limitations.

- It didn't kill you then, it doesn't have to keep hurting you now.

- You may have allowed past pain to create a habit of negative thinking. You are easily capable of programming yourself toward a much more positive attitude and outlook.

- First it is a choice then it is a matter of exercise to create the new habits, 'burning new pathways' of positive thought processes in your mind.

Person or Event	Emotion or Resulting Feeling

Person or Event	Emotion or Resulting Feeling

Once you have done this exercise, look at what you have written, realise that these things are distinct and separate from you. Take the positives if there are any to take (and there usually are), accept who you are because of it and you still have a right to peace and happiness in your life, then let it go. A good way of doing this is to throw it away physically, burn it in a kind of ritual ceremony, share it with others and then push it away from you mentally, physically and emotionally. You can do this and it does work. It may take a few repetitions as a lot of new habits and attitudes do take time to develop. It cannot remain a destructive force in your life if you have no need for it and give yourself the permission to be released from it.

Now why don't you take a few minutes to write down the positive things, the chance meetings and other lucky breaks and gifts that have come your way in your life. On the table overleaf you can record these occasions. This will help you realise that things usually balance themselves out in the end. You may have been much more fortunate than you think because you tend to remember the sad stuff and forget some of the good. We have all had triumphs, wonderful experiences and been downright lucky in the past. Take some time to write down any that you can remember. It will definitely cheer you up and remind that the past isn't all bad; on the contrary it was probably better than you remembered it.

Event or Lucky Break	Its Effect on You

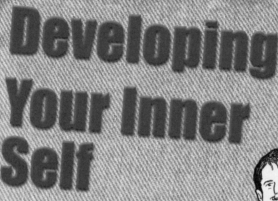

Developing Your Inner Self

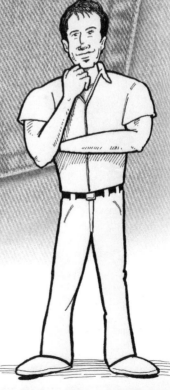

SENSE AND SENSIBILITY

Our senses help us to understand the world around us and its effect on us. The more powerful and developed our senses become, the more aware we are and the more information we have to make the best choices for ourselves. We have such a broad range of sensibilities and are in no way limited to the five basic physical senses that most of us believe to be the limit of our awareness. We have all heard about the existence of our so called 'extra senses'. With our intuitive powers, danger instincts, sometimes premonition-like dreams along with the potentials of memory and imagination, we have a much greater awareness than we think; potentially, that is, as always we don't always use what we have.

If we want to access these extra senses, become more aware and, as a result, be more powerful, we have to develop and tune ourselves accordingly. This book teaches you how to do this by becoming more tuned mentally, physically and emotionally and more knowledgeable of your capabilities. In this section we are going to talk more about our hidden senses and how actively to develop them. When we learn to use our hidden senses more, we become aware of the many levels the world and our experiences exist on (remember the different perspectives and mindsets we were discussing in the section on 'Black and White Thinking'. This in turn provides us with more information, which in this world IS power.

To begin with, we all know we have our basic physical senses of sight, smell, hearing, taste and touch but we also have many other subtler senses. These include **intuition, imagination, danger, purpose, scale, contrast, direction, intent, connection, truth, justice, rhythm/timing, balance** and **humour**. We use these every day to make up our full sense of reality. We just have to learn how to develop them more fully so they can become more of a tool. There certainly is more to life than meets the eye and when we are healthy and strong and have a fulfilling and stimulating lifestyle, we tend to get more out of a given experience or situation. This is because we have more powerful senses and are therefore aware of more things going on around us and on more levels. I would like to use a simple piece of scientific knowledge to help me explain what I mean by different levels and the whole picture that they combine to create.

Everything in our physical world exists on one level or another of what we call the 'electromagnetic spectrum'. This spectrum is the way science describes the different types of energy that make up the world as we know it. So, the energy spectrum represents the limits of the world we inhabit and our understanding of it. Like our creative process it has seven basic levels (these are, from lowest to highest vibration: radio waves, microwaves, infrared waves, visible and audible, ultraviolet waves, x-rays and finally gamma rays). We are used to believing that we are only sensitive to what we can see, hear, feel, smell and touch but we may also be aware of all seven of the levels, or at least many more than we are taught to believe exist.

Think of this energy spectrum as a radio set and then think of our minds and its senses as the receiver that we use to tune into the stations of our choice. The main station is chosen for us because of the fact that our normal range of awareness is that part of the spectrum consisting of visible light and audible sound. However we all know that things have more to them than a visible image and audible sound. As previously stated, we are capable of tuning our minds so that we have a broader range of 'stations' available to us, all providing their own type of information. If we take a movie as an example, we see the moving pictures and hear the sounds but there is a lot more to the production than meets the eye. There is a story, a script, there are actors and other props in each scene, there is the performance itself, there is the intent on the part of the filmmakers as to what the film is trying to convey and then there is the effect on the viewer. So we see and we hear the film but our overall experience of it includes so much more. However we can only speak for our own experience, what it did for us, meant to us and how it affected us. Two different people might have two totally different views on it and sometimes you can watch the same movie twice and see so much more the second time because you are more aware and therefore more informed as to what is going on.

What is important to understand from all this is that at any one moment we are tuned into our world and our world exists on more levels than just those that meet our eyes, ears and nose. When we are more fully developed and our powers are maximised we get more out of a situation or scene in our lives. This is because our extra senses tell us the intent and purpose, judge the quality and performance better, see its consequences and potential dangers or benefits and generally give us more information. So being more aware is invaluable to us in so many ways. It's nice to know at least you'll get more out of movies and music in the future. Train yourself a bit more and you will definitely get more out of life as little, if anything, will pass you by unnoticed. You will be a sensory powerhouse!

I believe it is vital for us to become more fully aware. After all it is very difficult to lie to or deceive an informed, knowing and sensitive mind. A more developed human race in the future will not so easily be sold inferior products or policies because they will be able to see through lies more clearly, detect the true intent of the seller, understand their effects and consequences and choose a better way or idea. At the moment we take too many things on face value and accept and consume far too many things that are bad for us both individually and collectively. The truth is there to be recognised, we just have to tune into it more thoroughly by using all of the senses we possess, not just the obvious ones. They are all there waiting for us, we just need to turn them on and tune in to them. With a fitter, well fed and relaxed body, a balanced, informed and focused mind, coupled with a loving and positive attitude, we are naturally more aware than we are without these strengths. So power up and uncover the layers of life that were previously hidden. Then you will become the master of your destiny and have so much more control over your life.

YOU VIRTUOUS DEVIL, YOU

Wouldn't it be nice to be more naturally courageous, patient, compassionate, enthusiastic, confident, purposeful, passionate and peaceful? Maybe you already are but if, like pretty much everyone walking this earth, you lack one or more of these virtues and would like them in your life but don't consider them to be part of who you are, think again. These virtues are aspects of the human ideal that we can all develop. We all have them lying latent somewhere in our psyche but, because we don't practice the things that we need to be this way, we don't get the benefit from them in our daily lives. Most of the time we have them to some degree but lose them under pressure or forget to use them or get run down and lose the personal power which fuelled and maintained them. We are all extremely virtuous entities but we must be relatively strong to have them as an asset.

You know there were times in your life when you had one or more of these in abundance but now they seem to have left you. Or you may have developed better patience and perseverance as you got older, wishing you had these qualities when you were younger and needed them more. Just like our different mindsets, they are all there waiting for you to develop and utilise them. As with all our other powers, physically, emotionally, mentally and creatively, these are ours to use, if we can bring them out through the development of our whole selves. The first step is to realise their availability and the next is to bring yourself back into balance and develop the strength holistically so that you do rediscover your virtues. Then of course comes the practice.

You may say that you don't have any patience but have you really taken a good shot at improving your stress levels and inner calm or actually practised having better patience during tough situations? Every day we are presented with opportunities to be more virtuous.

 Try practising using one or more of your virtues on one given day and then change it for another day and see how you get on.

In addition use your daily affirmations as a mental exercise, reminding yourself that you do have this virtue or that virtue, e.g. "I am brave, patient and creative", and support this mental exercise with your physical ones and your healthy eating plan. Remember, the more you actually use your powers, the more they become you and you, them. You may not have always been the most calm, patient, thoughtful, giving, brave, creative and honest person before but you can be now, you virtuous devil, you.

MAY THE FORCE BE WITH YOU

We all need spiritual as well as mental and physical stimulation. More than that, we need to have a spiritual aspect of our lives to ensure that we do not become materialistic and selfish. It is not more important to our immediate survival but we do need a healthy spiritual life to feel happy, content and secure.

We all know we are not going to live forever and this is a frightening prospect for many. So, to feel a deeper sense of comfort than we can get from careers, homes and savings, we all need to find faith and security in something with more permanence and meaning. We need to feel inspired that our life has purpose and what that purpose is. We need to have the ability to find peace in troubled times and never have to suffer despair because we have that inner strength and knowing that, ultimately, we will be OK. There is definitely more to us than just a body. It is this soul or life force that yearns for more in our lives than satisfaction and interest for our animalistic personality. We are often reminded that man cannot live on bread alone and it is with this in mind that this section exists. Any recipe that helps us reach our potential must include ways to satisfy our spiritual needs. Here is a recap to remind you of what they are:

Your top ten innerself needs

1. **Love** – It's what we live for, isn't it? Love, not money makes the world go around. When we care for and love ourselves, then we are open to love and be loved by others.

2. **Appreciation** – Learn to appreciate what you have; everything is a gift.

3. **Truth** – Be honest with yourself and others – you will be rewarded. ' Stand in your own truth and you will be empowered.

4. **Freedom** – Don't get tied down too much. Alongside your health, your freedom is your greatest asset.

5. **Laughter/Fun** – Be light and don't take life too seriously. Try to laugh and have fun every day.

6. **Inspiration** – It fuels our desire to live life to the full with purpose and excellence.

7. **Forgiveness** – We need to let our negative painful emotions go by forgiving ourselves and others for their mistakes. Our health benefits tremendously with the regular use of forgiveness and detachment. Grudges and regret are extremely harmful to your health and happiness.

8. **Nature/Beauty** – Food for the soul. The fact that we can appreciate beauty at all shows us we are beautiful ourselves. All of Creation is beautiful in some way and everything is connected.

9. **Communication** – Speak from the heart, don't hold in your feelings. Listen to yourself. Your heart and your conscience are the voice of your soul which knows you best and what is best for you.

10. **Challenge** – If life were so easy, we would shrivel up and die. We all need challenge to give us something to work towards, something to be passionate about and to hone and sharpen our senses and skills.

In addition to these we need:

- **Faith** – A feeling that a higher power has our best interests in mind.

- **Justice** – Fairness for everyone. If we live a good, honest life, we want to know that we will get what we deserve.

- **Camaraderie** – Friends, family and support.

- **Art** – Music, literature, poetry, we need all kinds of creativity to help us properly to appreciate life in all its beauty and diversity.

- **Nostalgia** – It is important to remember the good times.

- **Giving** – Remember the vital balance of give and take.

- **Beauty** – It is in the eye of the beholder but we all need it. The world can be a very ugly place at times.

- **Romance** – Don't be afraid to dream and be romantic.

- **Creative Expression** – It is a natural urge to be creative. It is energy we all have but it must be expressed.

- **Home/Roots** – To know where we come from and a good strong platform from which to operate and look forward to returning to.

- **Cooperation** – We have to learn how to cooperate with people as well as our environment.

- **Reverence** – Respecting and appreciating the important things, our own as well as other people's.

- **Aspiration** – Our natural desire to improve ourselves and our world. Don't lose this drive.

- **Passion** – Keeps us going, brings out the best, as well as sometimes the worst in all of us. Brings out our individuality.

- **Celebration** – Life is a gift and we must celebrate it when we can. After all, our days are numbered.

- **Guidance** – We all need to give and receive a little of this from time to time.

- **Solitude** – Take time and don't be afraid of time alone. We are born alone and we die alone.

- **Confession** – Get it off your chest, within reason.

- **Counsel** – Share your worries and give succour when needed.

- **Grieving** – Don't keep it in, let it out when you are upset or have suffered a loss. It will come out sooner or later.

- **Frivolity** – Be a little silly sometimes.

- **Escape** – We all need to get away from time to time. This may come from a movie or a trip somewhere or even just a book.

This is the full list of needs for emotional and spiritual contentment. Again appreciate what you already have and try to incorporate into your life what you are missing. Learn to be more loving especially to yourself. The happier you are the more you have to give others.

 Take care of yourself well and everyone around you benefits.

Not all things spiritual are religious in nature

We sometimes confuse spirituality with religion. This is a common yet very limited perspective. We are all looking for that feeling of calm, confidence and security, a meaning to life, a higher purpose, and a way of escaping the inevitability of death and taxes. We all need to feel loved, we need to care, we need to feel connected to things and to feel that we are not alone in this world. Religions are designed to help us get there, get connected, feel safe, feel loved and help us develop a faith in our lasting nature. Appreciation of why we are here, appreciation of our gifts and blessings, inspiration towards being a better person and a determination to live a loving purposeful life are all goals that religions try to connect us to and in most cases they are very reliable in doing this.

However effective religions can be, it is possible to get these feelings of guidance, inspiration and faith in an everlasting nature from sources other than religion. It has just been traditional that we follow one faith or another because these are systems already laid out, like educational and motivational courses. In the past we didn't have the leisure time or strong individual consciousness that we do today to find our own way. People nowadays are not necessarily following the faiths of their parents or even their culture.

There are many religions and faith systems available to us today and it is up to us to decide which one suits us best. The one key thing that we do need to find is the aspect of ourselves, an aspect that already exists, one that is never afraid, is always aware of our powers, is in touch with the Creative Forces of the universe and the part of us that always has compassion and acceptance of other people no matter what their colour, status, gender or faith. Mainstream religions and faiths still have a very important role in society. They help us stay connected to our purpose and deeper selves and they inspire us to be good, loving and compassionate people. We just have to be really careful that, in following these paths, we are not separating ourselves from others because our faith might be different from theirs (another example of black and white thinking). Religion should make us more loving, connected and accepting, not narrow minded and exclusive in our attitudes.

Spirituality is everywhere; we just have to tune in to appreciate it. We can learn to make spiritual connections anywhere and at any moment, we just have to see and appreciate things on a deeper level. When we are more spiritually developed we have better intuition and a better sense of justice, we are more purposeful and we come from a stance of love, acceptance and compassion rather than judgment, status and personal gain. A healthy spiritual life ensures we don't get too bogged down in materialism and selfishness.

Our futures on this planet depend on our ability to coexist harmoniously with our fellow man, our environment and to live sustainably. When we ignore this, problems start. We have to get away from the idea that this physical existence is our only reality. Not all things real are available to our five physical senses, we have already seen that. For much of life to be appreciated, we must develop this immaterial, spiritual nature. If we stay narrow minded in our physical, five sensory view of the world we miss out on a whole lot of life, and most of the best bits too. What is wealth without health? What is status without love? What is gain without security?

Sometimes we get so materially oriented that we reject the idea of God or a Creator because we have no proof and without proof we can't believe and appreciate or connect with it. It is important to know how alive the invisible world is. Everything is ultimately energy at the invisible, subatomic level. Science has shown us that it is only when this energy is concentrated, condensed and formed into patterns that it becomes a physical object, and something has to make that formation (or at least imagine it) to create the pattern in the first place (we do this in our own small way by the creative process explained earlier).

As we gain more knowledge of our universe, it has become apparent from our experiments that, its age, size, physical laws, the amount of matter within it and its concentration are all made possible by some very fine tuning. A decimal place here or there, a very slight difference in percentage of one thing over another and none of this would be possible. The sun wouldn't burn as bright or as long, would be too hot, too cold, there would be too much or too little gravity. No sun, no people, it is as simple as that.

Whatever it is that made all this possible, we are inevitably indebted to It and at the mercy of It, Him or Her. At the heart of our spiritual experience we need to feel a connection with the ultimate Source of all we know. It is this God, Creator, Source, Force, Overmind, Nature that we need a relationship with for us to be truly satisfied and balanced. The concept is general and Its form is for us all to make up our own minds about. One thing is for sure, we did not make ourselves or our world, we are just here now and able to experience and make sense of it with the minds that we have.

There is an unfathomable Force and Intelligence that has made all this fine tuning, physics, beauty and form possible and we should be in awe of what that is and what it means to us. Whenever we forget this higher power and place ourselves at the centre of the universe we quickly become unstuck. As I said at the beginning, we never have all the answers. Sometimes we just need to get back in touch with our ancient Source and ask for help. When we do and have faith in that Intelligence we always find the right way illuminated. Whether we believe or not, it is most likely that we have all have felt this guiding force in action at some point or another. We learned in the mind section that we are connected and sensitive to the full energy spectrum. Whatever is at the Origin or Source of this energy is connected to us, our bodies and our minds.

Through meditation and prayer we can make this connection and, when we do we feel all the security, comfort and knowing that we are looking for from this aspect of our lives, this capacity is there for all of us at any time.

As I said before, it is just a matter of tuning in and appreciating it. As long as we maintain a healthy spiritual life, we will always have this to draw from and the faith to give us strength and hope. We need to stop worrying about our differences and which religion is right or not or which race or gender is the stronger and get back to focusing on and enjoying our personal relationship with our origins and purpose. Our spirituality is a deeply personal thing and we have no right to judge the validity of another person's faith or inspirational source. Whatever story or inspiration resonates with us is what we need to focus on and enjoy. This will enable us to concentrate on being the best, most loving person we can be. The others we may reject or not need but it doesn't mean that the different connections other people make are necessarily wrong. We don't know how effective they are and how another person feels. We should learn from religions not to be judgmental and accept people for the quality of their characters and deeds.

There is no single right way or path but there is a single Creative Force and this is what we need to connect to and concentrate on, not whose story or culture is best or more right. If you feel it, you just feel it. If it makes you want to be a better person and gives you a true feeling of comfort even in times of despair, then it works. Life is about finding a way that works. The most balanced, healthy, sustainable and satisfying way to you is your right way. Life is still about fulfilling your needs and realising your potential and then living in a creative and harmonious way. So don't sweat the small stuff and always keep an eye and a place in your heart for things spiritual and purpose orientated. You might just find heaven here on earth. Anyone can add a little spirituality to their lives. Again it comes down to how you spend your time. You don't even have to leave home. Some examples of spiritual activities include:

- Church and religious materials

- Appreciation of nature

- Art galleries and listening to music

- Time with family and good friends

- Inspirational speakers/seminars, books or tapes

- Inspirational movies

- Meditation or prayer

- Yoga or martial arts practice

Whatever gets you there is up to you.

Having a spiritual life including things like going to church, giving to the community or charities, mentoring and volunteering, helping animals, brings out the better, more inspired and considerate person in us. Our self-esteem and confidence is fed by the love, appreciation and inspiration we get from maintaining a strong spiritual existence. We are animals by nature and driven to survive, procreate and satisfy our desires. Yet we are equally creators, good Samaritans and enthusiastic and cooperative communal livers. We have to get away sometimes from the take, take, take rat race and this is how we transcend the mundanity of the daily routine of bills, roads and concrete of our modern world and get back to something core and primitive. It comes in so many forms. Just make sure you devote some time to this aspect of your personality.

RULES FOR BEING HUMAN

1. You will receive a body. You may like it or hate it, but it will be yours for the entire period of this time around.

2. You will learn lessons. You are enrolled in a full time informal school called Life. Each day in this school, you will have the opportunity to learn lessons. You may like the lessons, or think them irrelevant and stupid.

3. There are no mistakes, only lessons. Growth is a process of trial and error and experimentation. The failed experiments are as much a part of the process as the experiment that works.

4. A lesson is repeated until learned. A lesson will be presented to you in various forms until you understand it. When you have learned it, you can go on to the next lesson.

5. Learning lessons does not end. There is no part of life that does not contain lessons. If you are alive, there are lessons to be learned.

6. 'There' is no better place than 'here'. When your 'there' becomes a 'here' you will simply obtain another 'there' that will again look better than 'here'.

7. Others are merely mirrors of you. You cannot love or hate something about another person unless it reflects to you something you love or hate about yourself.

8. What you make of your life is up to you. You will have all the tools and resources you need. What you do with them is up to you. The choice is yours.

9. The answers to life's questions lie inside you. All you need to do is look, listen and trust.

10. You will forget all this.

PEOPLE COME INTO YOUR LIFE FOR A REASON

People come into your life for a reason, a season or a lifetime. When you know which one it is, you will know what to do for that person. When someone is in your life for a REASON, it is usually to meet a need you have expressed. They have come to assist you through a difficulty, to provide you with guidance and support, to aid you physically, emotionally or spiritually. They may seem like a godsend and they are. They are there for the reason you need them to be. Then, without any wrongdoing on your part or at an inconvenient time, this person will say or do something to bring the relationship to an end. Sometimes they die. Sometimes they walk away. Sometimes they act up and force you to take a stand. What we must realise is that our need has been met, our desire fulfilled, their work is done. The prayer you sent up has been answered and now it is time to move on.

Some people come into your life for a SEASON, because your turn has come to share, grow or learn. They bring you an experience of peace or make you laugh. They may teach you something you have never done. They usually give you an unbelievable amount of joy. Believe it, it is real. But only for a season!

LIFETIME relationships teach you lifetime lessons, things you must build upon in order to have a solid emotional foundation. Your job is to accept the lesson, love the person and put what you have learned to use in all other relationships and areas of your life. It is said that love is blind but friendship is clairvoyant.

I thank the people who have been part of my life whether for a reason, a season or a lifetime.

SO WHAT NOW?
MAIN CONSIDERATIONS

Wow, we certainly have covered a lot of ground. Life is, after all, extremely complex, dynamic, yet at the same time really quite simple when it comes down to it. We have covered a fair amount about who we are, what we need to be our best, how to overcome our limitations, how to get strong and how to make the most of what we have. So after a short recap, I want to consider one last question and that is: What are you going to do with your new powers when you get them (if you haven't already) and how is this going to affect you and the world around you?

Recap:

Remember the seven phases of the creative process? Well, with the seven matching aspects of ourselves coming up, I intend to leave you with something simple and compact that you can use as a consideration of the big picture of your personal development. These will be your seven main areas to concentrate on when trying to improve your powers and heal yourself. There is a lot of information and instruction in this book and, after all, life can be really complex, as we have seen. If you stick to these seven main considerations as you move forward into your new tomorrow, you will be in a better place to keep it all in focus. This should keep you from becoming overwhelmed by the task ahead.

Your considerations for improvement are:

1. **PAST/ORIGINS** – We are the sum of what makes us; our parents, our ancestors, the earth, the universe, right the way to the beginning of time. It all had to be the way it was for us to be the way we are. There

is NO changing the past, but we do need to understand and appreciate ours better and reconcile what we can.

2. **OUR NEEDS AND DRIVES** – There is no getting past the fact that we are living organisms and animals and, as such, we have clearly defined needs to be well and happy. Know your needs better and you will know yourself.

3. **OUR CHOICES/LIFESTYLES** – What we do with what we have determines what we will become. Spend your time and resources wisely, be prepared and organised if you want good results in anything.

4. **NATURE/WELLBEING** – It is vital to know what is good for you and to make sure that you make this the focal point of your life, to do what is best at all times. Live sustainably, love and give through a natural desire to be as good a person and as natural a human being as possible. Is your life sustainable and geared toward wellbeing?

5. **COMMUNICATION/LEARNING** – Educate yourself, develop understanding, communicate clearly and honestly and stop to listen more. Improve relations with yourself, those around you and the environment.

6. **INTUITION/IMAGINATION** – Learn to trust in your inner vision and conscience. You have many hidden powers. Become physically, mentally and emotionally fitter and feel these grow and expand until you are full of love and light, creativity, compassion, yet immune to lies, deceit, greed, fear and negativity.

7. **FUTURE** – Surrender yourself to the future. There is no point in worrying about it, what will be will be. The only control we have over the future is what we choose to do and think today. Try to be your best at all times and there is no need to fear the future, or anything else for that matter.

Have a bit of fun along the way too!

I have worked with people from all walks of life from professional athletes and sports stars to doctors, lawyers, teachers and policemen through to school children and youth programmes, the elderly in nursing homes and even my own family (probably my toughest challenge). Whatever the problem or goal, I have always used the same formula which is the blueprint behind all of the LifeShaper programmes. When we are healthy and living a balanced and purposeful life, we look, feel and express ourselves in our best light.

Thanks for letting me be your life coach.
I would love any feedback and will answer any questions I can. Just email me at
lifeshaper@hotmail.com

Pete

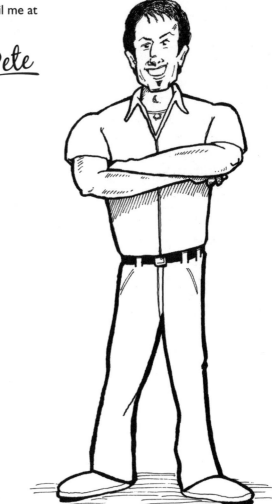